With These Hands

With These Hands

Maureen Fenner

Heartland Publishing

First published in 2002 by Heartland Publishing Limited
P.O.Box 902, Sutton Valence, Maidstone, Kent ME17 3HY
www.heartland.co.uk

ISBN 0 9525187 3 2

British Library Cataloguing-In-Publication data

A catalogue record for this book is available from the British Library.

Typeset in Adobe Caslon 11/14pt
Book design by Jeff Horne
Photographs from Ms Fenner's family collection

Printed and bound in Great Britain
on acid-free paper from sustainable forests
by The Cromwell Press, Trowbridge.

For Emma and Lucy
– and Tom

introduction

I am often asked how I manage to do certain things, from "How do you drive your car?" to "How did you pick up your babies?" So I decided to write this book, which contains the answers to both those questions and many more.

I contracted polio at the age of three months. I am able to walk, but a puff of wind would blow me over. My arms are completely paralysed, as is my left hand. I am able to use the fingers of my right hand and I wear a strip of elastic around my right wrist so that, when I want to raise my arm, I hold the wristband in my teeth and lift my arm with the strength of my neck.

This method of using my arm has proved a great success but, as with many simple solutions in life, came about by accident. When I was a toddler and wanted to lift my hand, I would bite at the sleeve of my clothing. As you can imagine, the sleeve would soon tear, so my mother began putting a band of elastic webbing around my wrist, and I have worn one ever since. Despite its simplicity, it has been the most important aid in my life.

Yet, although it is such a necessary aid for me and I have used it for so long, I am still somewhat embarrassed by using it in public, because of the attention it draws to me. But I am never without my strip of elastic, night or day, for to be so I would feel as though my arm had been amputated. In one way or another, almost every bit of independence I have been able to achieve, I owe to it.

In this book I will tell you about my achievements so far, and what I would still like to accomplish. I know as I go through life that, among a majority of 'normal' people, my disability will always attract attention to me. Drinking tea or coffee through a straw, for example, brings strange looks my way. Although, given an alternative, I would not choose to do this, it is preferable to having the drink spilled down my clothes, which is terribly humiliating and often a side effect when someone is trying to feed me. Besides which, I don't want to be fed; I am not a child.

And the way I write, by holding the pen in my mouth, always causes people to stare in sheer amazement as I sign after using my credit card in shops. The most common things that people say when they see this are "Oh, you are clever, how long did it take you to learn to do that?" or "How marvellous, you write better than me!" It's almost as though they look upon it as a party trick, or some kind of magic, rather than just a necessary method of writing for me.

There's no answer to any of these outpourings, so I usually try to ignore them and concentrate on what I'm doing, it being far more important to me that I write neatly because people don't expect me to be able to. I see it as part of my lot in life, the alternative to hiding away because I am different and because I don't do things in the same way everyone else does. Something which, you will appreciate as you read this book, would not be in character for me at all.

Over the years, I have hardened somewhat to these public situations, a necessity which I believe comes with maturity in order to cope with severe disability. It is also important to see the funny side of things, as people are sometimes very funny (usually when they don't mean to be).

For example, there was the man from a delivery company who, after delivering some goods to my home, handed the pen to me, not realising I couldn't take it with my hand. When I took the pen in my teeth and proceeded to sign my name he became very hot and flustered and said, "Oh, put anything dear, put Donald Duck if you like!"

"But that's not my name!" I replied. He was so embarrassed! I've come across people who assume I'm illiterate, and they do have to be put right. Like the woman who said, "Just put an X, dear." I told her that X is the mark of an idiot and continued to sign my name. She was far more uncomfortable than I was! Thankfully, I have been blessed with a sense of humour which helps me greatly when encountering such attitudes.

I should say at this point that it was my original intention not to disguise the names of any of the people in this book; I owe a great deal to so many of them and would like to acknowledge that. However, at my children's request, I have made one exception and changed the name of their father.

I have now told you something of my circumstances, so I'll go back to the beginning of my story.

one

I was born in Ashford, Kent on the 2nd of May 1955, the second child of William and Joan O'Sullivan. My sister Lynne was then eighteen months old.

My father was from County Cork in Ireland. He was a very handsome man with jet black hair and lovely green eyes that sparkled when he smiled. He met my mother during the war when he was in the RAF and she was in the WRAF. They were stationed in Egypt, in a place called Habbania.

At the end of the war they came to Ashford, my mother's home town. My father got a job in the railway works, which at the time were the biggest employers in Ashford. He started off there by sweeping up, and at first took lots of stick for being a 'Paddy', but he became an engineer and worked there for many years. By the time he left, he was greatly respected.

My mother was very pretty with black curly hair and blue eyes. I always remember the bright red lipstick she wore and the smell of her face powder. My birth was uneventful, and for the first three months of my life I was a healthy baby.

However, in the August I became ill with what was at first diagnosed as pneumonia. I had a severe fever, and within a few days it became clear that I had the polio virus. At the time there was a polio epidemic in Britain, but the vaccination against the virus was not available at the time of my illness. One of my life's great ironies is that the vaccination was discovered later that same year.

Once it was established that I had polio, I was admitted to hospital and put in an oxygen tent to aid my breathing. My limbs were bound with bandages to help prevent any further spread of polio through my body, as movement helps to stimulate the virus. Of course, as I was a tiny baby I had been moving and wriggling constantly, and because of the misdiagnosis the paralysis was already widespread.

My breathing had become laboured and it was usual for patients whose respiratory system had been impaired by polio to be placed in an iron lung. This looked like a large metal cylinder, into which the patient was placed to help the breathing. Thankfully though, when the virus finally left me, my respiratory system was undamaged, although both my arms were paralysed, my legs were affected and my spine was curved.

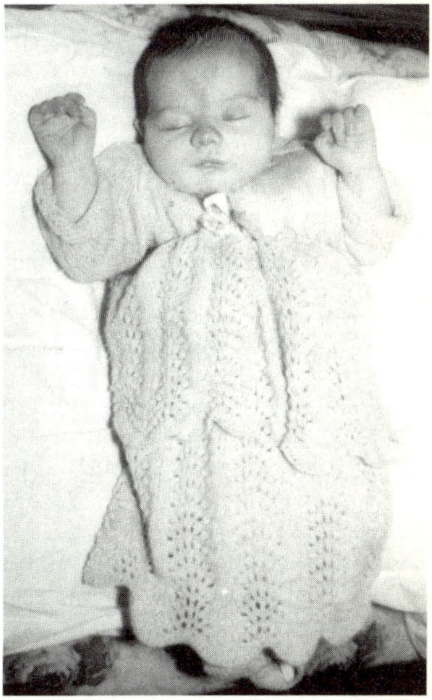

Three weeks before polio struck

For the next three years I was in and out of hospital in Ashford for physiotherapy and examinations. During that time I had my first operation: my left foot had 'dropped', which means it hung down because the polio had weakened the muscles, and the operation was done to fix my foot in the normal walking position.

When I was old enough to be mobile I began shuffling along on my bottom in order to get about. We lived in a three-bedroomed council house in Twelve Acres, a cul-de-sac in an area of Ashford called Willesborough. My parents loved me very much and were very attentive to me; I can remember being carried on my mother's hip as she did household tasks such as cooking, cleaning and anything else she could accomplish with one hand whilst holding me. I had a head full of black curly hair and big green eyes, and my mother used to say I was like a 'big dolly'. I suppose I must have looked like a rag doll at times, as my arms were completely flail.

I became very close to my sister as obviously we spent a lot of time together, and that closeness has remained throughout our lives. As far as my father was concerned, to me he was God. He would pick me up in his great strong arms and cuddle me. Sometimes, he would tickle me and I would giggle so much I could hardly breathe, and his loud Irish laugh would fill the house. Other times he would carry me out into the garden in the evening and we would look up at 'Mr Moon' surrounded by his beautiful stars. I was totally fascinated. My father would hold both my tiny hands in his great spade of a hand to keep them warm. I was absolutely happy at these times, I felt so safe. Nothing could touch me then.

It must have been heartbreaking for my parents to realise just how helpless I was. They were only in their twenties, and neither of them had had any prior experience of disability.

When I was two years old, my brother William James was

born. My father was ecstatic at having a son, but I was not best pleased at the arrival of 'Willie James', as he was known, and the joy his birth had created. My mother could no longer spend so much time carrying me about; there was a baby in her arms, someone else to focus on as well. When my father sat me on his knee, there was a baby on the other one. I became a very jealous little girl. On one occasion, I had been placed on my parents' bed along with my baby brother, and my mother's attention was distracted momentarily. I wasted no time in doing my best to kick Willie James off the bed, desperately wanting rid of this intruder! My mother was naturally horrified when she realised my objective and I can remember my severe reprimand. All I wanted was to have my parents to myself.

My sister Lynne, on the other hand, had never seemed a challenge to me in my parents' affections; maybe this was because she was already there before I was born, and she was very loving to me. My mother used to put me and my brother into a big black pram for my visits to the hospital or to take us

With my sister Lynne (right), 1958

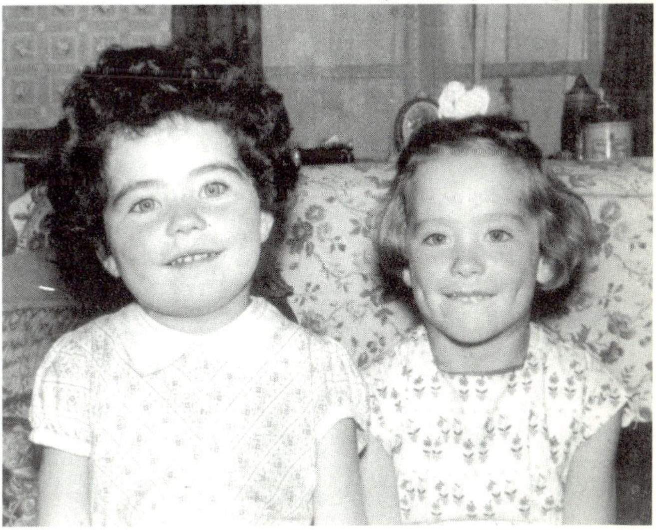

to the park, where I would shuffle around on my bottom. I enjoyed picking the daisies and giving them to my mother, and once she had shown me what a daisy chain was, I wanted to wear one forever. I became furious if the chain broke!

I still had regular hospital appointments; as well as physiotherapy I would have electrodes strapped to my arms to try and stimulate the muscles into life, but this turned out to be a waste of time.

Because I was known to the hospital, the Social Services became involved in my situation, and thoughts turned to my long term future. Obviously, I wouldn't be able to attend school in the ordinary way; I was three years old and unable to walk or do virtually anything for myself, so plans had to be made. Oblivious to my many problems, I was happy enough. As time progressed, I became more used to my brother's presence, and once he was able to sit up and play I thought rather better of him, as long as he didn't get more attention than I did!

At the age of three I was of course completely unaware that there was anything wrong with me—I was in a loving home and all my needs were catered for. However, things were going to change dramatically; a decision was going to be taken that would change my life and that of my family forever. My world was about to be blown to pieces.

two

It was decided by the authorities that I should leave home and go to a boarding school-cum-hospital in Sussex, some sixty miles from Ashford, called Chailey Heritage Craft School and Hospital, which treated children with all types of disabilities.

My parents took me there for the first time on 11th November 1958. I thought it was great when they sat me down on the floor to play with the toys and the other children. It was Poppy Day, and I remember there was a table to the side of the ward covered with a white sheet which enhanced the brilliance of the bright red poppies for sale. Absorbed in play, I was vaguely aware that my parents were talking to a short plump woman with dark but greying curly hair, wearing a uniform. She turned out to be the ward sister, and her name was Sister May.

I was not unused to nurses' uniforms, having already spent a lot of time in hospital, so I wasn't unduly bothered by their presence. It was not until some time later, when my parents kissed me and said "Goodbye" that I had the first notion that I was not going home with them.

I watched in horror as they walked away, leaving me in the arms of Sister May. I can still remember the panic rising in me, and crying out as feelings that I had never experienced took over. I was utterly devastated; I could not believe it. Where had my family gone? Who were these people? What was this place? Where was I? Had they forgotten me? Why hadn't they taken me with them? I was three and a half years old and I couldn't ask these questions—I just cried and cried. I was put in a metal cot. I could see out between the bars of the cot side, and I remember how cold the metal felt against my damp face.

The ward had cots down either side; the floor was covered with brown linoleum and the windows had metal frames. There were two enclosed cubicles in the ward, painted white with big windows. One was the sister's office, which was in the centre of the ward. There was another cubicle at the far end of the ward and, when my cries and screams would not abate, this was where I was wheeled in my cot. I was told by a nurse that I could come out when I stopped crying, as I was upsetting the other children. I spent many days in the cubicle.

Naturally, some memories are blurred after so many years, but I can remember the emotional agony, the forlorn hope every day that my mother and father would walk into the ward and take me home. I felt as though I had a heavy black block in my chest weighing me down with sadness.

The nurses were not unkind, though their manner was brisk and efficient. There was no place for kisses and cuddles at Chailey; it was very much a regime. The days were of strict routine, which was necessary in an establishment like that. I remember that there was a small black and white television high up on a shelf in the corner of the ward which we were allowed to watch for a few hours during the day. For some reason, I came to believe that the lady who I saw regularly on the television, who was in fact the Queen, was my mother! I think this was because, like my mother, the Queen had short dark curly hair and wore red lipstick. So whenever the Queen came on the television I would inform everyone "there's my mummy"! Needless to say, I got some very strange looks from the nursing staff, while the other children on the ward just looked at me in amazement!

Another thing that I was convinced of throughout my childhood, was what God looked like. In my mind's eye, God was a very short man, who wore a large black cape and a flat checked cap! He also wore very large dark glasses, like sunglasses, so that I could never see his eyes. Where this image came from originally, I have absolutely no idea!

The ward I was living on at this time was called the Queen Elizabeth Block, known to everyone there as QEB. It had been opened by the Queen Mother some years earlier. There was an outer section to the ward, which had brick walls and large metal framed doors opening on to a concrete area outside. Our cots were put out here on winter evenings, as it was believed that fresh air was good for us, and we were told this often by the

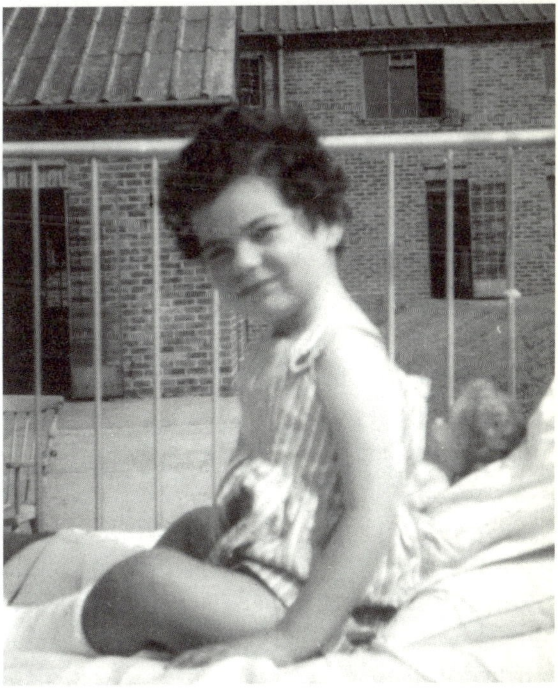

In my cot, outside Chailey, 1959

nursing staff. Some of these 'fine' evenings, however, were also very cold. During the summer and autumn months we slept outside, and were not brought back into the ward unless it actually rained. Our cots were protected with burberrys, thick canvas covers with very rough edges.

Having no alternative, I became accustomed to my new life over the next few months. Gradually, I stopped spending every day staring at the door hoping my parents were coming back for me.

That Christmas of 1958 I spent at Chailey. I learned years later from my mother that Sister May wrote to my parents, saying I was settling down well and it would be a shame to disturb me by letting me go home for Christmas. I didn't see my family again until late January. Oddly, my memories of that meeting are very blurred, but obviously it must have been tremendously emotional for both myself and my family.

Around the time of my fourth birthday I had an operation on my left hip to insert a metal plate. This was screwed into my hip joint, to help give me more stability so that I might be able to walk. Shortly after the operation I was fitted with a calliper, known as a 'short iron', which went from my knee down. The purpose of this was to support my left foot, and stop it dragging and tripping me up, as the previous operation I had at the Ashford hospital had not been particularly successful. I then began sessions with the physiotherapist: at first just standing independently, then slowly progressing to taking a few steps.

My physiotherapist was Mrs Pearson, a cheery soul with pure white hair and a ruddy complexion. She laughed a lot, and I warmed to her straight away, affectionately christening her 'Mrs P'. She gave me great encouragement, because I was terrified of falling over, especially as I wasn't able to use my arms to hold on to anything like crutches or a walking frame. I much preferred to sit down at every opportunity that became available. If I could get near to a wall, I would lean on it and slide down onto the floor, so that I was safe.

As my walking became more proficient, Mrs P and I went for short walks around the grounds. I would hold on to her finger with the little strength I had in my right hand and she would tell me about her children and her home in nearby Lewes. One day Mrs P brought me a Red Indian doll. It wasn't very big, and it had come free inside a packet of washing powder, but I treasured it and it accompanied us on our walks, its head poking out from Mrs P's pocket. I remember a huge water tank in the hospital grounds with metal steps leading up to it; when I asked her what it was, Mrs P told me it was where she ate her sandwiches, and being none the wiser, I believed her for ages! On the whole, though, I didn't really enjoy walking as, unavoidably, I often fell quite heavily.

I began walking on the ward, which was even worse. As soon as I had recovered from a fall and had any wound stitched or swabbed I would be stood up, away from a wall, and told to start again. My tears and screams of real terror were ignored by the nursing staff, and I just had to get on with it. Often my head and face were badly cut, and it was suggested by the senior doctor that I should have some protective headgear made to save my head from the impact of these numerous falls. This 'helmet' was similar to what boxers wear when they are training and I hated it, not least because the other children used to laugh at me, and I knew it looked silly. Being so young, I had no appreciation of the damage that might be sustained to my head as the result of continuous heavy bumps, and since my arms were flail I was totally unable to break the fall.

I had made friends among the other children with whom I lived so closely. We were, after all, in the same boat, all there because of some disability. Each of us had been separated from our families; indeed, some had been abandoned by families who felt unable to cope with a disabled child. These children had no visitors, and nothing to look forward to; they went without the emotional comfort that comes with belonging to a family, being a part of something, really mattering to someone.

three

OVER the next few years I had more surgery, including operations on my right hand to strengthen my fingers: I had a bone removed from my left arm, which I could not use at all, and put into my right wrist, which gave me greater use of my right hand. The surgeon who operated on me was Mr Donal Brooks. A much respected orthopaedic surgeon, he worked mainly in London hospitals and came to Chailey about once every three weeks, always on a Saturday as that was the only day operations were done. Mr Brooks would arrive in a large chauffeur-driven car which would be parked underneath the trees in the hospital grounds. I would stare at its shiny bodywork in awe and wait for its passenger to come in and, as he often did, encircled by the doctors and nurses from Chailey, sit me on his knee and explain what operation he would perform next to help me.

Children who were not being operated on that day would be seen in his clinic before Mr Brooks began the surgery. There he would check the outcome of previous operations he had undertaken, or see other children who might benefit from surgery in the future. He was a very gifted surgeon, and helped me a great deal with his expertise. By the time I left school, I had undergone some 25 operations on my feet, hands and arms, as well as surgery on my left hip to increase my stability for walking.

Chailey Heritage consisted of three sections: New Heritage, Junior Dormitory, and St George's. New Heritage, which was where QEB was situated, was a site with four other wards: there was a babies' ward; Tidemills, where boys and girls lived from about six years old; a boys-only ward; and Rennie Ward, for girls only. Children were admitted to these two latter wards at about the ages of nine to eleven, at which time they were segregated. The nurses' home was also on this site, as was the main kitchen and staff dining room; the operating theatre; the recovery room adjoining the theatre, where you were taken after surgery; the physiotherapy and X-ray departments, a Chapel and a sewing/laundry room.

As I grew older I was moved from QEB, where children from about two to five years of age lived, to Tidemills Ward, which was a few hundred yards away. Schooling on Tidemills Ward became more earnest. The teachers came onto the ward each day, and if we had recently had surgery, we had our lessons from our beds just as soon as we were sufficiently recovered.

I enjoyed school here. As soon as I learned to write I began to do so by holding the pen in my mouth; at first I had been discouraged from doing this, as it was hoped that the surgery I had undergone would enable me to hold the pen in my hand, but although I was able to write in this way, it was so much easier and instinctive for me to take the pen in my mouth that after a while I was left to my own devices.

My last move within New Heritage was to Rennie Ward when I was nine. Some children who were profoundly disabled would remain here for the rest of their time at Chailey, usually until the age of sixteen. These children might have spina bifida acutely; this could mean they were doubly incontinent and unable to have surgery to help with this. In some cases, girls with this disability had an operation to pull a section of their bladder out through their stomach; they would then have a rubber bag fitted over the section of bladder, which they could empty when necessary and thus cope with their problem independently. But this option was not always possible, especially if the condition was complicated by mental illness or hydrocephalus, known as 'water on the brain'. In these cases they would have an operation to insert a valve to drain the water off. Many of these children had enlarged heads because of their condition, and not all these children survived.

Other children had severe cerebral palsy; they were not able to control their movements or speak audibly and would always need round the clock care. Thankfully, although my condition was severe, improvements in my abilities had been made during the time I had been at Chailey so far, and the surgery had given me some independence.

I had also begun having occupational therapy, which was helping me in learning alternative techniques to do things for myself, such as going to the loo, dressing, washing and generally looking after myself. My occupational therapist's name was Jill Rockey; she was an extremely kind person who had a great understanding of the problems which faced me. Over the years I spent at Chailey we worked together to overcome many of my difficulties, and became great friends. As I was not yet very old the issue of my independence had only been touched upon. However, it would be concentrated on to a far greater degree as I grew into adolescence.

By now I was going home to my family regularly for holidays three times a year. Although I loved seeing everyone and being at home, my brother and sister had their own friends, and of course I didn't know anyone outside my family. My walking ability was improving constantly, though I still had to watch

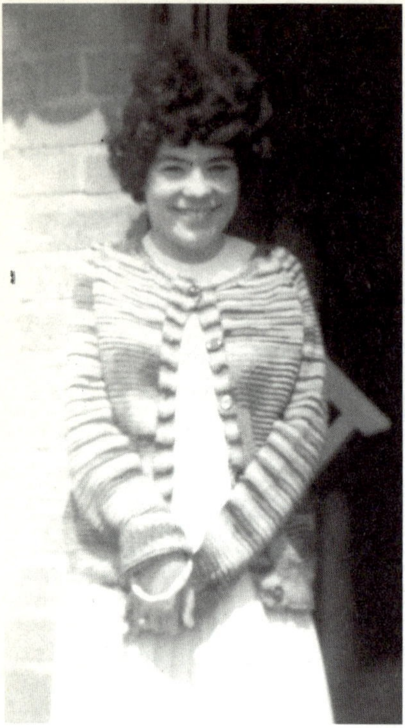

Summer holiday at home, 1963

every step I took so that I didn't trip over. Unlike the attitudes at Chailey, which was just to get on with it, my family were as terrified of me falling over as I was. For this reason, I didn't walk very much outside my home. I remember one occasion, though, when I wanted to show off my walking skills and was going confidently round the block with Lynne holding my hand. The pavements were uneven flagstones, and I tripped over and cut my head. My parents were mortified, and I interpreted their reaction as anger. In fact, they were just dreadfully upset to see me like that, but I remember thinking that I wouldn't walk much while I was at home, not wanting to upset them again.

When I was six my sister Anne was born, so my mother's hands were full. Lynne always did her best for me though. I had a big black pushchair which I could still fit into, and she would take me out in it to the shops or to the chip shop. I particularly remember her taking me to the local post office where they sold children's dress rings. Lynne would park my pushchair outside and go in and ask if she could bring the tray of rings out for me to choose one. I loved their bright colours and used to take ages deciding which one I wanted. After poor Lynne had taken every ring out of the tray and tried it on my fingers, I would usually buy a red one which I would wear until it fell apart! Sometimes Lynne would bring her friends into the garden and we would play 'The Man From U.N.C.L.E.' This entailed Lynne and her friends being secret agents and rushing around looking for clues, while I was Mr Waverley, the boss who sat at his desk and gave the orders!

My brother and I got on a little better by now, although he was always trying to get control of my pushchair. When he did finally achieve this, he would run with it (and me) as fast as he could, with no thought of uneven pavements or kerbs. I lived in dread of being tipped out but luckily I never was, and these episodes were kept to a minimum thanks to the vigilance of Lynne and my mother.

Sometimes, though, I did play happily with him. On one occasion I suggested we take the family goldfish for a ride in his toy lorry. I instructed Willie James to lift the goldfish out of its bowl, and place it in the trailer of the lorry. From there he pushed it up the garden path, the fish's tail wagging in despair as the poor thing gasped for air, and I shuffled along on my bottom singing the theme to *Wagon Train*, a cowboy programme on television at the time. When the fish finally became still I gave it a prod with my finger, and realising there was something seriously wrong, suggested we return it to its bowl before we were found out. We were of course found out, when the fish was seen floating on top of the water in its bowl, and my brother and I were duly told off!

On another occasion during the Easter holiday one year Lynne and I went to the shop in order to buy Easter eggs for friends. We bought about eight altogether and stopped off in the park on the way home, where we started talking about the friends that the eggs were for. One by one they were discussed and their qualities brought into question, and during the space of less than an hour we had eaten all the eggs, having decided between us that the friends we had bought them for weren't really nice enough to warrant the gift anyway. Needless to say, we both felt quite sick!

I was now being taken back and forth to Chailey by a member of the Social Services, and although parting from my family was still dreadful, I got over the worst of the tears once the initial goodbyes had been said and I was on my way. We often picked up a boy in Tenterden on the way back to school and he used to bawl his eyes out as he was prised away from his mother—which would start me off again. We endured more emotional suffering than children should know about.

four

When I was eleven I was moved from the largely medical environment of New Heritage a few miles down the road to Junior Dormitory. As the name suggests, here we slept in dormitories rather than wards. Junior Dormitory itself was a huge old house in which boys and girls lived if they were ambulant. The dormitories were upstairs and we had our meals downstairs in the dining room; the kitchen was also on the ground floor, as well as the television room and the sister's office. As I was unable to manage the stairs I was carried up and down by a member of staff.

A few hundred yards away from Junior Dormitory was the school site, with proper classrooms and teachers specialising in different subjects. There was also a church which the Church of England children attended every Sunday and Thursday mornings. Being a Catholic, I was taken back to New Heritage on Sundays where Mass was held in one of the staff conference rooms. I wasn't very happy at all at this stage of my life; I hated the fact that I couldn't manage the stairs and most of the other children could, albeit with crutches or just by holding on to the banisters.

I think this was when I started to realise how disabled I was, being with children who were quite a bit more mobile than me. Of course by now I knew I was different to 'normal' people, but my life was still very sheltered, so the degree of my disability wasn't always apparent to me. However, having no alternative is a great reason for getting on with things, so that's what I did.

I found the schooling side of life stressful, especially in the mornings when we had to line up in the playground before going into assembly in the Hall. The playground was presided over by Mr Holgate (who of course had the nickname Colgate), who would shout really loudly if we were not all standing still, lined up and quiet before filing into assembly. The problem for me was that there was a step about five inches high around the edge of the playground, which I couldn't manage, so I had to leave the line and walk to a different part of the playground where the step was more shallow.

The first time I did this, Mr Holgate's voice boomed out across the playground, "Maureen O'Sullivan, where do you think you're going?"

I carried on towards the smaller step; all eyes were on me during this episode and I wished the ground would swallow me up. My total concentration however, was on getting up that step, a height of no more than two inches, without tripping up and falling flat on my face in view of the whole secondary school. When I had successfully achieved this, I walked back to where Mr Holgate was standing—his face seemed to have taken on a purple hue by this time—and explained exactly what I was doing, at which point he calmed down and gave a slight nod in the direction of the assembly hall. I carried out this same routine during morning line-up for the rest of my school days and hated it on each occasion. I think it's worth mentioning that Mr Holgate had himself lost a leg in the war and wore a false one, so he didn't exactly sprint along either. I guess he felt at one with us at Chailey Heritage.

The place was also sometimes called 'The Public School of

Crippledom', though this title had been more widely used when the school was founded in the late thirties by a nurse called Grace Kimmins, who was later made a Dame for her work.

The teachers were for the most part a kindly bunch, and sometimes they were very funny. There was Mr Field, the Science teacher: he was in his forties, with a balding head that would turn bright red as he shouted for quiet in the class, which could be raucous when we were all yelling at each other. He was not the type of teacher that instilled any fear into us, as his kindly face would break into a smile as silence reigned. He had been a Major in the Army so he had the nickname 'Maj'—or 'Osram', because his head resembled a light bulb! He was a sweet man and I liked him a lot.

Then there was Miss Dennis, who taught Domestic Science. With her we made cakes and bread, and occasionally cooked whole meals to which we could invite anyone. Sometimes we had to wash the aprons in a twin tub washing machine; I found this very laborious, especially dragging the washed aprons out of one tub and pushing them into the spin drier on the other side.

As far as cooking was concerned, even though I only had the use of my right hand I could do quite a lot. I could mix the flour and butter to make cakes so long as the bowl was held steady, which was achieved by placing it into a specially cut out ring in the table. The only thing I couldn't manage was putting things into the oven. We also had to wash up all the things we had used; Miss Dennis was a stickler for things being done perfectly, and she had a brash tongue if she wasn't pleased with our efforts. She was in her late forties, a well-built woman with grey curly hair and a frequently dripping nose. She walked with her back and shoulders slightly forward and her bottom sticking out; she would put her hands behind her back and her handbag would swing from her fingers back and forth as she walked along. She was a heavy smoker and would often be overcome by a fit of coughing; and as her face grew ever more cerise in colour, I would wonder what we should do if she died in front of us in the classroom.

One of Miss Dennis's sidelines was stamp collecting. She started holding a stamp club during the lunch hour, and those children who were interested were invited to bring any unusual stamps along. I must confess I have absolutely no interest in stamp collecting, but one lunchtime when it was raining hard, I took refuge in the Domestic Science room and attended the stamp club. We sat around the table, Miss Dennis at its head, and about five other children watching as she carefully laid out stamps from countries all over the world, talking about each stamp in turn. Suddenly she was taken over by a coughing fit and the stamps were blown all over the table and some on to the floor. A look of fury crept over her face and she tutted loudly through her spasm of coughing. I roared with laughter at the spectacle, I had absolutely no control, and as I am unable to put my hand over my mouth to stifle my laughter it rang out loudly over the classroom, in competition with Miss Dennis's coughing. When she was able to speak, she shrieked at me to get out at once, and said what a stupid girl I was. I left the classroom still overcome by laughter: that memory still makes me smile. Miss Dennis and I were not the best of friends after that!

Other lessons I had included Art and Maths. Art lessons were fairly unremarkable as I have no talent in that area, but Mr Pinner, a tall, slim man with a receding hairline and a bushy beard, was kind and we used to laugh a lot in his lessons. I have always loathed Maths and I'm very bad at it. Our teacher, Mr Pollard, was a short stocky man with a northern accent, who would shout at you if you didn't understand what he was endeavouring to teach. He would often get worked up and single one pupil out, making them stand up in class (even if it took ages!) so that he could make a spectacle of them. Overall, I received a comprehensive education at Chailey, with English being my strongest subject.

I was also instilled with a great deal of discipline, an integral part of the Chailey regime. Everything was done strictly by the clock; lateness for meals or lessons was unacceptable and would be punished either by being sent to bed early or having privileges withdrawn. This was very deeply felt by the child concerned, as privileges were few and far between at the best of times, but watching the hour or so of television allowed or staying up a little later at the weekends would be denied any child who broke the rules at Chailey Heritage.

The final stage of life at Chailey was the move to St George's, when I was about thirteen. It was a large, monastic-looking building situated about half a mile from Junior Dormitory. It had four different wings which housed either boys or girls up to sixteen years of age. The dining room was huge, with wooden tables placed in rows along either side; the kitchen adjoined it and the food was brought out on trolleys and served from huge pans. At St George's we slept in dormitories of four and were looked after by wardens. There were fewer nurses, as at this stage most of us had been given the medical treatment we needed; now getting each of us as independent as possible by the time we left school at the age of sixteen was the main objective.

Our lives were controlled by the ringing of the bell, telling us where we should be and thus what the time was. The first bell rang at seven o'clock to get us up in the morning, and breakfast was at eight o'clock. I was still having occupational therapy and could wash and brush my teeth independently, and I was now even able to dress myself partially. My school uniform, which consisted of a blue blouse and grey skirt, had been sewn together and a long zip had been put down the centre. By hanging it over the back of a chair I could sit on my bed and step into it, and sort of wiggle my arms into the armholes; then I would bend down and grab the corner of my blouse in my teeth to pull it off the chair on to my shoulders and zip it up, all of which left me quite exhausted for a while. I could never manage my socks, so I could have help with them, and my tie was on elastic. However, I was working towards independence.

After breakfast, the bell rang for inspection so we all had to be by our beds, standing if possible, and the Head Nurse/Matron would walk up one side of the dormitory and down the other, checking our appearance for school and that our beds and lockers were tidy. As soon as inspection was over we headed for school.

St George's was rurally situated, with common land surrounding it. Those children who were able had to walk the half mile across the common to school; there was a concrete path halfway down but the rest was just grassland, although it was kept reasonably well cleared. It was decided that on fine days I had to walk to school, but I could take the school coach otherwise. I hated being lifted on to the coach because the gentleman who usually did this was very elderly with warts on his face, and I dreaded being close to them.

Once aboard, I would be picked on by the older boys, because at that stage of life my hair was quite unruly and I found brushing it very difficult. A member of staff sometimes endeavoured to do this for me, but the tangles were very painful. I had been given the nickname 'golliwog' because of this; my hair was regularly pulled by the older boys and I was quite helpless to stop them. It was dreadful—some of these boys were aggressive, and thought nothing of punching and kicking the younger, more defenceless children. So although I was worried about walking across the common to school in case I fell, sometimes it was preferable to taking the coach.

At this time I had my first crush. His name was Doug and he was one of the four drivers at Chailey. He was some twenty years older than me, not particularly handsome but very kind, and he always had a smile for me. He had been married, and had the reputation of being quite a flirt with the nurses. I didn't care about his reputation though—I just thought he was lovely. As time progressed and there were two coaches to choose from to take us to school, I would always do my best to get on the one he was driving, as near to the front seat as possible!

When I was fourteen I began using a special typewriter, with a method known as POSM (Patient Operated Selector Mechanism). This involved me having a plaster cast made of my right hand, with spaces for my fingers cut out so that I could move them up or down. Into these spaces microswitches were inserted, and I had to learn a code of finger movements,

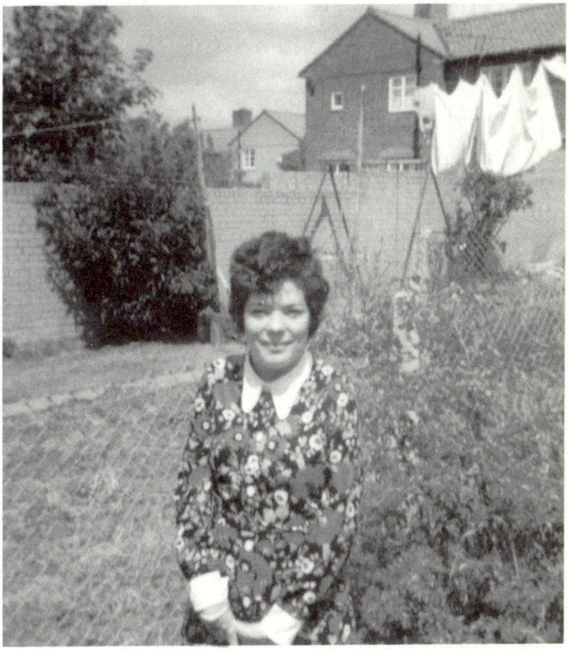

At home in Ashford, 1968

combinations of which made letters. For instance, if I touched the microswitch above my right finger twice I would get the letter 'd' and if I only moved the same finger once I would get a different letter. It sounds very complicated, and it was, although once I had learned the code and completely memorised it, which took me many weeks, I attained an acceptable speed. The typewriter was positioned on a trolley, and underneath it on a lower shelf was the 'brain' into which my movements were transmitted and deciphered into letters.

It was also possible to operate the typewriter with one's breath. By holding a tube in the mouth, and sucking and blowing in various combinations, letters could again be made. I never tried this method myself, but I am sure that for people who have no use at all in their limbs, it was a great alternative. With POSM controls it is possible for very disabled people to open and close doors and curtains, operate light switches, use computers and carry out many other such everyday tasks, giving them a much treasured independence.

I would spend every lunch hour in the classroom practising, and was very pleased to have a legitimate reason to stay in at lunchtime, as I had always loathed the playground where the children had to go once they had finished eating. I was not able to run around like some of the children, so I used to stay near the wall where I felt more confident. I was quite a noisy child, always shouting at my tormentors to leave me alone, but really what other defence did I have?

As I grew older and the time to leave Chailey drew nearer, so did my fears of being in the outside world. For thirteen years I had lived a very sheltered life, nowhere near to a town, and apart from the staff and the visitors who used to tour the school on what we called Zoo Days, we saw nobody. We did go out on school trips sometimes, to places like the Tower of London, and there were annual outings to the Ideal Home Exhibition and Littlehampton Amusement Arcade, where we used to get free rides all day. However, these journeys were obviously very well planned and we were looked after by the staff, so it was nothing like real integration with the public.

When the time came for me to see the Careers Officer, I was so worried about being in the big wide world that I said I wanted to be a nun! I did go to church, but I wasn't what you'd call devout by any stretch of the imagination. As I had been given the training with the special typewriter, it was logical that I should take up some kind of secretarial training when I left school.

Each Christmas at Chailey, a Nativity Play was put on by the children. It took place in the church, with a tableau of the Nativity being put on in the cloisters. Those cast in the tableau had to keep as still as possible as Friends of Chailey and visitors filed into the church and gazed at us. I was once cast as an angel, and being the giggler that I am, found it very hard to look angelic. Later, in my final school year, I was cast as Mary in the Nativity Play, which was very enjoyable, and we always had a real donkey in the procession both in and out of the church. It was very moving at the end of the Play as we filed out of the church and the organist played *O Come All Ye Faithful*. In my final year however, the donkey disgraced himself on the way out of the church, right in the middle of the aisle. While I suppose it added to the authenticity of things, George, who looked after the donkey, was most embarrassed!

In the summer of 1971, after thirteen years, I left Chailey Heritage. Although I had been through some harrowing times there, I believe that I was given the best medical attention I could have asked for. My physical capabilities had been stretched to their utmost, and I had a level of independence far greater than most people would have thought possible, given my severe paralysis. My walking was as good as it was going to get and although I still fell sometimes, my falls were now far less frequent. This was largely due to the fact that as I grew older, I took more care, hardly ever taking my eyes off the pavement as I walked, as the least thing would still trip me up. I had long since discarded the protective headgear; can you imagine the ribbing I would have been in for from the other children if I had worn that as I progressed through the school?

In spite of the hardships of my school years, my experiences would stand me in good stead for the future. I was sad to be saying goodbye to Doug; he had been so kind to me and the thought of seeing him had given me reason to look forward to the day. People said I would forget him very soon after I left school, but actually we wrote to each other up until I was in my twenties and, as you see, I never did.

five

I spent the summer of 1971 with my family. By this time I had two brothers and three sisters. My youngest brother, Davy Joe, was born when my mother was forty and I was fifteen; my father was absolutely delighted that he at last had another son.

Because I was now leaving school, Ashford Council allocated us a house with a bedroom and bathroom downstairs. It was also a larger property than my family had previously had and was situated within walking distance of Twelve Acres where they had lived. My older sister Lynne had by now started working at Kent Paper Company doing secretarial work, so I didn't see so much of her.

I spent almost three months at home before starting college. In October I went to Queen Elizabeth's College for the Disabled in Leatherhead, Surrey, where I was to do a course in shorthand and typing (my specially adapted typewriter had been brought home from Chailey).

My first impression of the College was that it was huge, and the classrooms were all quite a distance from one another. There were so many people there, from my age to middle age, and some of them didn't look outwardly disabled. After booking in, I was shown to the girls' residential block, Springbok House, situated about a quarter of a mile from the main offices and recreational facilities. There was a minibus which belonged to the college, adapted for wheelchair users to cope with the distances.

Once again we lived in cubicles of three or four, each cubicle sectioned off by a curtain. I was with two girls who had also been at Chailey, and one of them, Carol, was also doing the same course as me. She was completely independent in spite of having spina bifida and she used to help me with dressing. There were no nurses here, only one sister, a complete dragon called Sister Fareigh. The other girl who had been at school with me, Sheila, also had spina bifida, though unlike Carol she could not walk at all and her condition was far more acute. She needed more medical care than was available at college, and after a few weeks she became very ill and was taken into hospital. She did not return.

Our dining room was also in Springbok House, as was our classroom, and we had to be there at 8.15 every morning having had breakfast and looking presentable. Our tutor, Mrs Berry, was a short, dark-haired woman who would put up with nothing less than the best. If we made any mistakes while typing letters, she would point it out and roar "Not mailable!"

I endeavoured to learn shorthand, but found that the outlines and different thicknesses required were difficult to do with my mouth, bearing in mind that I was controlling the pressure of the pen with my neck, and it was unlikely that I would ever be able to build up enough speed to make it viable to employ me. Mrs Berry suggested that I try Speedwriting, which is really just an abbreviation of words along with a few dots and slashes. This proved more successful, and although it was not possible to attain the same speeds as when doing proper shorthand, I became proficient and acquired the RSA Certificate I worked for at the end of the course.

Queen Elizabeth's College was for both men and women,

and we did meet up in the evenings to socialise; this would be either in the main hall to watch a film, or at a club in the grounds where students could buy drinks. I had my first relationships there; it was my first real taste of teenage life outside the boundaries I had been used to, and at first I found so much freedom quite frightening. Some of the men there were married and doing courses as weekly boarders, returning home at the weekend. They would try their luck, sometimes not letting on that they were married, but I soon got wise to them! At weekends a lot of the other girls went home, including Carol, who lived reasonably near in Horsham, and then I did feel alone.

The college bus was available to take any students into the nearby town of Leatherhead, if they wanted to go, on Saturday mornings. This bus had a lift at the back for wheelchairs, so I was able to get on easily. When we reached the town centre, we were dropped off and I made my way to the post office. This was the first time I had been out on my own in my life. I remember walking along very hesitantly, scrutinising the pavement for anything that might trip me up. I could feel people looking at me; I do have a pronounced limp, and anyone who is in the least different draws unwanted attention. I was the proverbial fish out of water, totally unprepared for the outside world and as lonely then as I have ever been.

On reaching the post office, I leant against the wall in order to get up the considerable step into the building, as people pushed their way past me, and finally I joined the queue. When it came to my turn, my signature was required and as I took the pen in my mouth and proceeded to sign, the woman behind me who had been peering over my shoulder, said in a very loud voice, "Oh, you are clever!"

This caused the rest of the queue to look, and I felt as though the whole world was staring at me. I wished the ground could have swallowed me up there and then, I was so sick with embarrassment. I made my way back to the bus with tears streaming down my face, more conscious than ever of the fact that I couldn't even wipe them away. I felt completely ill equipped to cope with the world; in spite of all the positive things I had been taught at Chailey, integration into society had not been one of them. Maybe there was no way I could have been prepared for the onslaught of attention my disability would draw to me, but in retrospect I think that I should have been taken out much more during my later years at Chailey, and introduced into the world beyond its walls. I didn't venture out of the college again during the nine months I spent there, having been badly stung by my lone experience. I did go home for the Christmas holidays, but I didn't talk much to anyone about my experiences, feeling that able-bodied people wouldn't be able to understand.

I made quite a few friends within the college, however. One girl I especially remember was Wendy; she was paralysed almost totally, though she could move her hands a little. One afternoon our class were having our break outside on the lawn. There were about ten of us drinking tea and chatting, and Wendy was sitting in her wheelchair smoking a cigarette. A gust of wind caught her hair, blowing it against the cigarette. In seconds her hair was alight, and she could do nothing at all about it. Our screams alerted the kitchen staff, who came running outside, one of them smothered Wendy's head in his apron. I could see, as he wrapped Wendy's head up, that the side of her face and head were already burnt. The fact that she had peroxide on her hair made things worse. She was rushed to hospital and as the rest of us were left in a shocked silence, I shall never forget seeing pieces of her hair on the grass. Wendy had serious burns to her head, and her face was badly scarred, but she did return to college after some time in hospital. Seventeen is not an easy age for anyone, but when you have the hang-ups of adolescence, as well as trying to come to terms with a severe disability, it is especially difficult. I felt very frightened and wondered how on earth I would be able to live my life; I was as low then as I have ever been.

I was much more comfortable in the company of other disabled people; they understood something of my anxieties and I could relax with them. One disability that quite a few of the other students at college had was epilepsy. I had never seen anyone keel over before, as there had been no-one at school who suffered this disability, and the first time it happened I was absolutely terrified. One of the things that could trigger an epileptic fit in some people was the sudden flicker on and off of lights. As it was the time of the miner's strike, the lights would often suddenly flicker before a power cut, and it was quite common for someone to fall over and have a fit. I remember on one occasion being instructed to sit on this person who was having a fit, to prevent him from hurting himself as he flailed about. There were already a couple of people trying to restrain this poor man; I had no intention of joining in, so I made as hasty an exit as I could.

When I saw people who didn't have obvious physical disabilities after that, I gave them a wide berth, simply because I was frightened. This isn't so surprising really; their movements during a fit were very uncontrolled, they would lash out, and as I was unable to protect myself, I felt very vulnerable if I was near them.

I had a few driving lessons while I was still at college. I had expressed interest in learning to drive, and knew it was possible, as while I was at Chailey we were visited by a man who drove by steering with his foot. His arms had been paralysed due to polio, and I was sure that if he could do it, I could. The difference it would make to my life would be enormous, so I was delighted when told that I would be going for an assessment to drive a motorised tricycle. This was what was known in those days as an invalid carriage, a dreadful title for one's first car. However, if it was going to give me some independence I didn't care too much. What was far more important was the ability it would give me to go out on my own.

My instructor was called Fred, a very happy-go-lucky person with a balding head and a good sense of humour. The motorised tricycle was dark blue in colour, and was powered by batteries that were housed in the boot; it sounded like a milk float when it went along! Its top speed was fifteen miles per hour. On the floor was a metal disc, which had a bracket fixed to it into which I slid my right foot in order to steer. With my left foot I operated the foot brake, and the parking brake was situated on the floor between my legs: it had a metal loop on one end into which I hooked my finger so that I could pull it

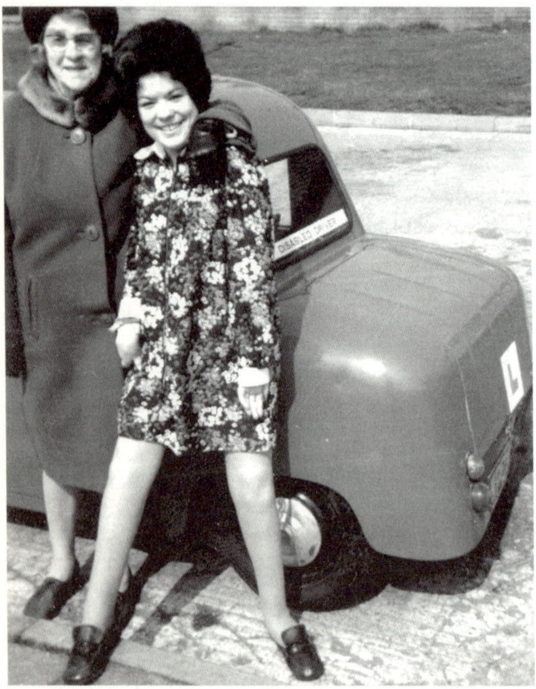

With my Nan and first three-wheel car, 1972

up to put the brake on. This was a bit tricky, especially when I was moving off after doing a hill stop. I had to really struggle to keep my balance while making sure not to take my foot off the brake, or the vehicle would roll back!

I was not required to take a driving test before going on to the road; I had a provisional licence. I thoroughly enjoyed my driving lessons with Fred. There was only one seat (mine) in the motorised tricycle, so Fred squatted down on the floor. As the door wouldn't then quite close, he tied it closed with string, leaving a gap from which his bum protruded! It was in this kind of hilarious situation that I learned to drive! Our route was usually the outskirts of Leatherhead to begin with, and I progressed to a few lessons in the town.

I must say that I wasn't exactly given a comprehensive knowledge of the Highway Code by any means, just the basics of driving the car, and the rest I learned by experience. The batteries had to be charged every night and topped up with water regularly.

I left Queen Elizabeth's Training College in the summer of 1972 having obtained the RSA certificate for which I had studied so hard. I was not sorry to leave, although I had made some friends there. I had been thrust out into the world and come face to face with my disability and its effect on the public.

I went home to Ashford, and my motorised tricycle was delivered shortly afterwards. The first time I drove the it to show my family, I forgot to take the parking brake off. The stench of burning rubber filled the air, and the car would not even reach its top speed of fifteen miles per hour! My parents were understandably nervous about me driving, but I was determined that I would do it. Even then, though, I would have much preferred a proper small car (four wheels are always safer than three).

The noise of the motorised tricycle didn't improve as I drove along. It was just as well the NHS didn't provide in-car entertainment—I would never have heard it!

I was visited at home by the Disablement Resettlement Officer (known as the D.R.O.), whose job it was to find work for me. Within a few weeks he set up an interview for me at a company called Proprietary Perfumes Limited, which made perfumes for many household items, together with flavours for toothpaste. They were looking for a copy typist to work in their typing pool. The interview went well, and the company arranged to pick up my special typewriter so that I could start work straight away. I remember the look of amazement on my mother's face when I told her I had got the job! She was of course delighted, as was my father; his face shone as he told me how very proud he was of me.

Although I was pleased that I had got a job, the thought of working with people staring at me all day filled me with horror. I kept imagining their faces as I used my wristband to raise my arm, or how they would stare at me as I walked with what was once described by a doctor as my "peculiar swinging gait"! But, as with so many things in life, the actual reality of doing something turns out to be less traumatic than the dread anticipation of what might happen, and after the initial month or so I felt accepted in my new job.

I drove myself to work each day in my little blue car. I hated the fact that these vehicles were known as invalid carriages, the word 'invalid' meaning 'of no value'. Disabled people are certainly not of no value, although sometimes the attitude of our able-bodied counterparts would lead us to believe so. This is why we have to be strong mentally, and believe in ourselves and our abilities.

Looking back on that motorised tricycle though, it really was the most horrendous thing to drive. Traffic would roar past me, and because its appearance was so different from the other cars on the road, it let everyone know immediately that I was disabled (which I couldn't care less about now, but in my adolescence was desperately important to me).

I worked in the typing pool with about ten women and a supervisor called Irene. She was in her late forties and wore brightly coloured blouses with large bows that tied under her chin. She was a kindly lady, but she fussed over me like a mother hen, which was suffocating at times. We took our work from a tray on Irene's desk; it consisted mainly of reports, letters and orders for materials used in the making of the perfumes. People from all departments brought their work in throughout the day, so I got to know who was who quite quickly.

On the whole, I found people to be friendly, and once the initial awkwardness of being new was past I settled down well. I knew, however, that Irene was protecting me from doing anything she considered to be too challenging, and this became quite frustrating, especially once I got into the swing of things. One of my frustrations was that I was only doing copy typing, and not being given the opportunity to use my speedwriting that I had worked so hard to master at college. Although I had been employed as a copy typist, I did hope that in time I might be allowed to progress to something more of a secretary. I made a few friends within the typing pool, and went out socially to parties and pubs now and again, though my friends were mainly in their early thirties and married with children.

I found living at home very different to what I had been used to. My father now had a car breaking business and his yard was a couple of miles from our home. His evenings and weekends were devoted to that, although he still worked in the railway works during the day.

My mother now worked at the nearby Energen factory for a few hours in the evenings, which she enjoyed as a means of

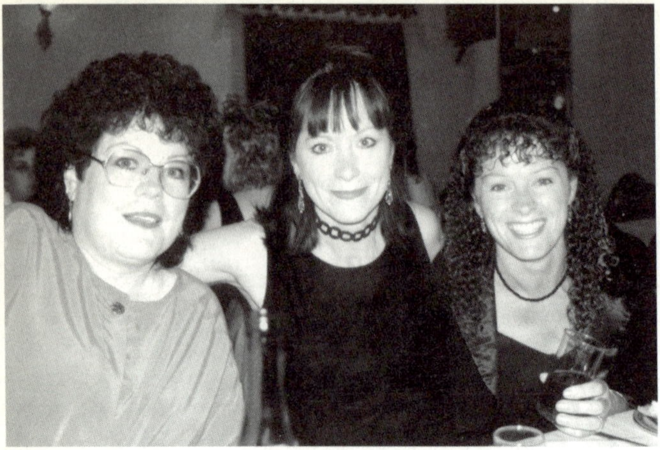

With Lynne & Catherine, much later in Ashford

getting out of the home environment as well as helping with finances. So I kept an eye on my younger sisters—Anne, who was about thirteen, and Catherine, who was nine—and my youngest brother Davy Joe, who was now three.

My eldest sister Lynne had by now left home and was living and working in London where she had a secretarial job, and she came home at weekends. My other brother Willie was sixteen or so, and always out on his moped or with his friends. I would usually sit and watch the television or spend time in my bedroom listening to records, and this is how my life carried on for the next three years.

six

AFTER a few months of driving to work, winter and the dark evenings crept up on us. On my way home one evening, I was hit from behind by an elderly driver, who succeeded in pushing my motorised tricycle into a ditch. Luckily, I was protected from injury by the batteries stored in the rear of the vehicle. This incident sapped my confidence, though, and I wasn't interested in driving it any more; I really wanted an ordinary car with foot steering put in. If I couldn't have that, I wanted the other type of motorised tricycle available on the NHS—although it was still a three wheeler, at least it had a proper engine, ran on 2-stroke petrol, and could reach a speed of about forty miles per hour.

My father, however, was not keen that I should drive again. He had been worried about me steering with my foot anyway, the whole concept being totally alien to him. I would often see him sitting in his parked van, waiting for me to pass a strategic point on my way home from work, such was his concern for me. Later, when he arrived home from his yard, I would ask him why he had been watching me, and he would reply that he just happened to be there at the time!

Now that I had been in an accident, it was arranged that I should be taken to work and brought home by a girl who lived nearby and worked with me. Although this arrangement solved the immediate problem of my transport to work, it left me feeling totally dependent on others, a feeling I loathed and battled with constantly. As the years passed, I became very depressed with the monotony of the routine, and desperately wanted to drive again. I also wanted to do something different, to stretch my abilities to their fullest, and I couldn't do it while I was living at home. I didn't want to cause my family any further worry, or to hear anyone say, "You can't do that Mo, you might hurt yourself."

I felt so trapped inside my body: I needed to achieve the ordinary things that people of twenty often want, like having their own space and having relationships, and I knew that to achieve these things, I would have to move away from home. It was so ironic—after all the heartbreak I had suffered as a child, because of having to be away from home, now as a young adult I wanted to leave; but as we grow and change, so do our needs.

My occupational therapist and great friend at Chailey Heritage, Jill Rockey, had helped me to overcome many problems with dressing, toileting and other aspects of personal care. I had always found her easy to talk to, as she worked with disabled people all the time and knew what I was capable of despite my disability; she didn't have the fear for me that my family had. They wanted me to be happy of course, but because of their love for me they were fearful that I wouldn't be able to achieve the things I wanted; that because of my disability I wouldn't, for instance, be able to drive again, which I was absolutely determined to do.

The trouble with other people's fear is that they can pass it on to you, and as you absorb it you begin to doubt what you are capable of as well. As you listen to their concern it plants little seeds of uncertainty into your head. You have to hold on very tightly to your belief in yourself; it's so easy to lose it. I didn't want the weight of anyone else's fear; obviously I was unsure of my future, but I knew I wanted change. So I took a few weeks off work, and went down to Cuckfield in Sussex to stay with Jill. We talked through how I was feeling: the urge that I had to move away from home and do something that I found interesting. I had secretarial skills, and that opened up possibilities for me, as typists were required in lots of different jobs. I was interested in the possibility of working within a hospital environment in a social work department, or with disabled people. I had no objection to living on the premises, as that seemed to me to be a good way of getting to know people.

Jill had heard about a possible solution to my problem. There was a residential home for the elderly, St Mary's House, situated on the outskirts of Brighton, and the matron was looking for a secretary. The position was for someone who would want to live on the premises.

I went along for an interview, with feelings of excitement as well as apprehension. I could see as soon as we pulled into the drive that it wasn't going to be access-friendly for my disability, as there were two steps at the front entrance. Once inside, we were greeted by the matron, whose name was Pat. She looked to be in her early forties; she had short hair and was wearing casual clothes rather than the uniform I had expected. She led us to her office, which was down three steps (and it had not escaped my notice that had we gone in the other direction, there were three steps to get up!).

Pat told us about St Mary's House, which was home to thirty elderly residents. It had previously been run by nuns, and although this was no longer the case it still had a religious background and all the staff were Catholic. My duties would involve clerical work as well as dealing with the residents' problems when necessary. My room was situated at the top of the house and there was no lift, so I had to decide whether I could manage the steps on a daily basis. I knew that I could get up the stairs on my bottom, but would only be able to manage that once a day; and I could manage the upper steps by leaning against the wall—although it would be by no means easy for me. However, it was an opportunity for me to leave home and get some independence, so despite the architectural problems, I decided to give it a try.

The wages were not very much but my bed and board were taken care of, so I knew I would have enough to live on. I returned to Ashford and told my family that I would be living away from home, explaining that I had become very bored with my life as it was and needed to have some independence.

On the whole my parents were quite understanding, saying that if things didn't work out I was always welcome to go back home. I did not go into great detail about the fact that there were so many steps around the premises, as they would only

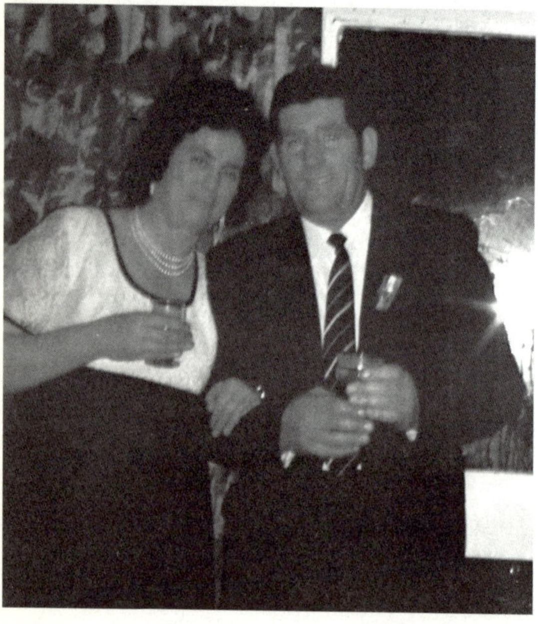

Mum and Dad, c.1975

worry and there was no point in that.

I moved into St Mary's House in January 1976. My room was very small but quite cosy. Because of the difficulty I had in getting upstairs, I soon got into the habit of staying downstairs all day, only going upstairs to bed. There were two other members of staff who also lived on the premises: Gloria was a few years younger than me and seemed very nice, and despite her youth was very self-confident and good with the residents; and Olive was in her early forties, mad about Omar Sharif and forever comparing lesser mortals to him!

Olive was also a manic depressive. Some days she would be on such a high, singing and joking, and other days her moods would be very black. During those times it was obvious from the glazed look in her eyes that it was a struggle for her to do anything at all. Sometimes she would just cry constantly, really sobbing and quite inconsolable. It was very hard for me to witness this because she was such a lovely person and would do anything for anybody. Quite often she helped me to get dressed in the mornings; her touch was so gentle, and she always worried that she might do something wrong and hurt me accidentally. Eventually her depressive state got the better of her and she took an overdose. She was found some hours later in her room and rushed to hospital, but sadly died soon afterwards. I will always remember her, though; she was a good person.

Gloria and I made friends straight away. She had a fine sense of humour, and shortly after I arrived she invited me out for the evening with her to a club in Brighton called Jenkinson's, where they had a resident band and a disco.

I thoroughly enjoyed myself; it was so good to be out doing ordinary things, and it didn't really matter to me whether I could dance or not—although in those days I used to get up and have a shuffle about, being very careful that I didn't get pushed over, I just felt so free to try things out without worrying anybody. We had a really good laugh, and at the end of the evening Gloria decided we would walk back to St Mary's, as it wasn't very far and she didn't mind pushing my wheelchair.

On the way home amidst our silly giggles we decided to stop and have a cigarette. I smoked in those days, mainly because it seemed like the right thing to do, but I can't honestly say I ever really enjoyed it. We stopped in a shop doorway, and had not been there for very long before we heard voices.

As they got nearer, I heard a man say, "Here they are!"

I looked up to see two men standing in front of us. I recognised them as I had seen them both earlier in the evening in the club. The older of the two had a not particularly attractive face, with slightly protruding eyes, skin which didn't look very clean, and greasy hair. He smiled to reveal a smattering of yellow teeth.

"Want a chip?" he beamed. Both Gloria and I declined his offer.

"I'm Barry, and this is Ken. We saw you in Jenkinson's and thought you wouldn't be far away."

Ken was in his early twenties, slim with receding brown hair and a beard. Although he smiled he didn't say anything. I thought he looked rather nice—certainly much nicer than Barry.

"Would you like a lift home?" continued Barry. Gloria and I looked at each other.

"What about my wheelchair?" I asked.

"Oh, that's no problem, we'll shove it in the boot." When you're young you don't worry about things too much, and bearing in mind that we had had a few drinks and I was getting rather cold, we decided to accept their invitation.

As Gloria pushed me towards where their car was parked, I said quietly to her, "I don't like yours much!" Ken then asked whether he could push my chair.

"Yes, if you want to," I said, feeling very relieved that it was not Barry who had made this request! Once we were back safely at St Mary's House, we invited Barry and Ken in for coffee, and they eagerly accepted. Barry made silly jokes, mainly I suspect to cover any embarrassment he may have been feeling.

Ken and I spoke a little; I told him what my work involved and that I had only just moved down to Brighton, and he told me that he had lived there all his life and his work involved making cash machines. After we had finished our coffee, I said that I was tired and going to bed, and thanked them both for the lift home. Ken immediately asked me whether I would like to go out with him soon. I was amazed—I had so little self-esteem in those days—but said that if he rang me we would arrange something.

Barry duly asked Gloria, who declined the invitation. I didn't blame her one bit, although I suppose I felt rather sorry for him.

Over the next few weeks I settled down into life away from home. Whilst my new job had been a way out of my rut, it wasn't quite as rewarding as I had hoped. Things moved along at a slow pace, and while I got on well with some of the residents, I found others difficult.

To counter that, however, I had the friendship of Gloria, and over the next few weeks Ken became very attentive to me. Most evenings he would come and take me out; he didn't drive, so he would push me down to the town in my wheelchair when we went for a drink. He had no problem with my disability—in fact I think he quite enjoyed caring for me—and our relationship grew rapidly.

In hindsight too rapidly maybe, but looking back I can see how it happened. Here was a good looking man who was obviously very fond of me, and for the first time in my life I was experiencing the ordinary things that people of my age did. Ken had recently moved out of his parents' home into a room of his own, which was situated at the top of two flights of stairs. His bathroom and toilet were on the first floor, which made it a very impractical place for me. However, as we got to know one another I began spending some of my free time there. It wasn't very far from where I worked, but unfortunately the room was also at the top of a very steep hill, which Ken used to push me up in my wheelchair. He would then carry me up to his room, which like my own was quite cosy, if rather small.

As I settled into my life in Brighton, I began to think about driving again. The only type of mobility I had at that time was my wheelchair, and as I relied on people to push it, I was totally dependent on others, a state (you may have gathered by now!) I am not comfortable with. I contacted the relevant department at Brighton General Hospital, and after a few weeks it was arranged that I would be assessed for a three wheeler invalid carriage again. However, this time I insisted on having the type that used petrol rather than electricity and would at least allow me to keep up with traffic.

My assessment was successful, and after a few months I was provided with a motorised tricycle which, after two or three lessons driving around the grounds of the hospital, I was permitted to take out on to the road. I did have a basic knowledge of the road, and as before, only required a provisional driving licence for this vehicle.

I always thought it a strange idea that one could never take a passenger in these trikes: it was as though the powers that be didn't think that disabled people had friends or family. I was delighted with my new independence, though, and while 40 mph was not going to break the sound barrier, it felt quite fast enough compared to my first motorised tricycle. As with my previous one this was very noisy, so again a car radio was out of the question! But that wasn't important to me, I had some freedom and independence, and I was happy.

When I went out with anybody I would meet them at our destination. Ken would take the bus or walk; it wasn't an ideal situation, but it was better than him having to push me everywhere. St Mary's House was proving to be a good starting ground for me; I was going out regularly, and in a very short space of time after leaving home I was in a relationship, something I had never thought would happen so quickly. Ken was extremely kind to me in those days; he didn't have many friends apart from Barry (who, it transpired, was married and didn't spend much time with him).

I gathered from what Ken told me that his life with his parents had been stormy. They didn't know he was leaving home until they actually saw him moving out, so communication was obviously not good there.

After a month or so of going out with Ken, I was invited to Sunday lunch at his parents' home. I was extremely nervous, as always when meeting new people. For instance, I can only use one hand, I need my food cut up for me, and if we have peas I need a spoon to eat them—all things which make you feel different and to which other people have to become accustomed.

Ken's parents had no experience with anybody who had a disability. I remember when I first met them, his mother spoke about me as though I wasn't there, and when Ken had carried me down the steps to their front door the first thing she said to him, over my head, was, "Nice looking girl Ken, isn't she?"

She was an unremarkable lady, who had brought up six children. As I talked to her I realised that she had a sentimental outlook on life, so whenever I tried to explain anything about my disability she would always say "ahh", which (at first) I found amusing. Ken's father was a small built man. He looked at me a lot on our first meeting but didn't say much; I thought he was probably wondering what his son had got himself into. I expect both his parents thought I was completely helpless—as indeed I am in situations where there are steps, and chairs too low for me to get up from independently, as was the case on this day. As I have said, Ken came from a large family and over the next few months I met them and got on well with them, feeling accepted and comfortable in their company.

As the months passed, Ken and I saw one another almost daily. Our feelings for one another had grown into what we believed to be love; we were never happier than when we were together, and one evening Ken asked me whether I would like to move in with him. I was delighted to accept his invitation, so I moved out of St Mary's House, although I continued to work there. This arrangement worked well, as it made life easier for me, even though Ken would have to carry me upstairs. The main problem we had was that the toilet was on the floor below our room, and in extreme emergencies I had to use a potty, which was very degrading.

We were very happy with our lives together though, and when, during the summer, Ken asked me to marry him, I accepted. We got in touch with Brighton Council and asked whether we could go on to their housing list for accommodation that was all on one level. As expected, we were told that there was a long list, so it could be some time before we were housed.

In fact it was almost a year before we were offered a two-bedroomed flat on the outskirts of Brighton. It was a spacious flat, situated on the first floor of a high rise block, but there was a lift. The area was known to be quite rough; there was graffiti on the walls as you entered the block and in the lifts, which also smelt of urine. It was in fact quite an eyesore from the outside, but it was our first real home together and we made it cosy, so we didn't mind. We had a balcony which looked out on to the racecourse and underneath was the car park. A parking space near the entrance to the flat had been allocated for my car, which meant that I didn't have far to walk and there were no steps at all.

Ken and I were married in March 1977, in St Mary's Church which was quite near to St Mary's House where I was still working. The staff there helped with the food for the reception which was held in a nearby hall. My mother and father were very pleased at my marriage and all my family came to the wedding. I was happy, I was 23 years old and looking forward to a life with Ken. We didn't have much of a honeymoon, as we just couldn't afford it, but we stayed for a few days in a holiday home in Hove, which was better than nothing.

During the time I had known him, I had noticed that Ken's temper had quite a short fuse. I realised that he was relatively new to helping someone with a disability, and these things take time to get used to. The main thing, though, was that I knew he loved me. He was a nervous man, and would sometimes stutter when speaking to people, especially people he didn't know. This happened in situations when the onus was on him to ask about something in a shop or speak on the phone, and once I realised that he had a problem I would do those things. He would also get flustered when he was packing the shopping in the supermarket, particularly if people were watching him, which was something he really hated.

When we had been married a short while I left my job at St Mary's House. The wages were so low, and now that we had bills to pay we needed more money coming in. Ken was still working at the cash machine factory and his wages weren't good either, so I went to an employment agency to find secretarial work.

The woman behind the desk looked at me as though I had been beamed down from Mars. I began to fill in an application form and noticed a pink hue rising in her face as she offered the usual "Isn't your writing marvellous! How long did it take you to learn that?"

I ignored her gushings, explaining that I had done it all my life, and tried to get across to her the practical problems involved in getting work. I needed to be able to park my car close to where I would be working, and I couldn't manage steps so it had to be flat. She said, in her best patronising voice, that she would do her best to find me work, but that Brighton wasn't the most suitable place as it was full of older buildings that had steps into them. From experience I knew that to be the case and didn't expect it would be easy to find employment for me—after all, nothing had come easily to me in my life. Even so, I was entitled to ask for help in looking for a job, and it was her job to help find me one.

The first interview I attended was at a solicitor's office in the heart of Brighton, but that wasn't successful because the toilet was outside. My second interview was with a finance company, again in the centre of town; I would be working with four other ladies doing copy and audio typing. Although there were two steps into the building and my car was a short walk away, I decided that perhaps this was the best I might get, so when I was offered the job I took it. The supervisor of the office was a woman called Betty; she was quite elderly and had been in the job for years, but she seemed nice enough and helpful.

We had to collect our work from a tray which was on Betty's desk; sometimes this was difficult for me, especially if there were a lot of separate pieces of paper to carry. However, I did as much as I could for myself; I didn't want to ask for too much help, particularly when I had just started there. I felt after a few weeks that I was doing well in the job. The only time I had to ask someone to do something for me was at coffee time, because the drinks machine was on the floor below our office, and I liked to have a hot drink. I didn't feel at all awkward about this, as one of the girls would go downstairs and bring up a tray of coffees for the whole office.

After six weeks or so, however, I learned that all was not well. It was a very windy day, the sort when I can hardly keep my balance to stand up, so I telephoned Betty from home and asked whether someone could keep an eye out for me and come to my car to give me a hand.

"Well, it's not very windy here," she said, "but we'll keep a look out for you."

There was an edge to her voice which indicated to me that she wasn't particularly happy about someone coming out to my car. I wasn't feeling very well that day and not very confident about going out. Since my balance is so poor, and as I am not able to hold on to anything for support, I am very vulnerable to falling.

When I arrived at work, nobody came out to help me, and it was all I could do to hold my car door open and get out. People take for granted using their arms for such a simple task as this, and when your arms are paralysed it's very difficult to cope. I finally got into the office, shaken up and angry. Able-bodied people can have absolutely no idea how it feels to experience such feelings of helplessness. It's really frightening to think you're going to fall, and worse when you know you can't save yourself or get up.

The atmosphere was heavy, and no-one spoke. I was furious with Betty, and once I had taken my coat off, I asked her why she hadn't sent someone to help me.

She didn't look up from her work as she said, quite casually, "Oh, we didn't notice you had arrived, we're busy today."

At that, I went along to the personnel office and told them what had happened. It was then that I was surprised to learn that certain ladies in the office had complained about having to fetch my drinks from the machine. I was extremely hurt and amazed at the selfishness of some people. Knowing this, however, I no longer had any wish to work there, so that day became my last in paid employment.

When I told Ken what had happened, he understood my decision to leave the job, and agreed that people like that are not worth putting in an effort for. And the reason I hadn't been feeling very well soon became apparent, as early in 1978 I learned that I was going to have a baby.

seven

BOTH Ken and I were delighted with the news, though we knew there were many struggles ahead. Initially however, I just wanted to savour the fact that I was pregnant. I felt so powerful, so normal. To me, my womanhood outweighed my disability by far. It was something I had always hoped would happen, and the reality of being a mother, of having another human being dependent on me, made me feel very happy. My parents and family were very pleased with the news, although I am sure they didn't expect me to be able to look after the baby myself. This, I would learn, was to be the common view. I remember someone saying that Ken would probably give up work, but this was not an option financially—and besides, even in those very early weeks of my pregnancy, I was certain that I would overcome the difficulties.

I knew these would be substantial, and that how I would achieve the many tasks ahead involved in the daily care of a baby, without the use of my arms, was as much of a mystery to me at the time as it was to anyone else. But my determination was strong that I would look after my baby myself. People would regularly ask me so many questions about how I was actually going to do various tasks—picking the baby up, feeding it, dressing it, bringing its wind up—and I didn't have the answers.

There was, after all, no blueprint for me to follow, and, apart from a girl at school who'd had polio, which affected her arms in the same way as mine and who used her feet (which were not affected) like hands, coping successfully with caring for her babies, there was nobody to ask. The only way I would find out how I would do things would be to try, and obviously I couldn't do that until the baby was born.

One thing I was fairly certain about, from very early on in my pregnancy, was that I would pick the baby up in my teeth, but I didn't say too much about that thought to others for obvious reasons! I could just imagine the panic that would spread across the faces of the recipients of my idea. "You'll drop it!" was the retort I was sure I would hear most often. Nothing other than the 'normal' way of picking a baby up in one's arms would enter the heads of people. That was natural enough, I conceded, but I simply couldn't do that. So I would do it differently, and I was sure I would succeed. But it would be no use debating this point until I could put it into practice.

The first three months of my pregnancy were uneventful except for the common morning sickness I experienced, but just after this I began to have some bleeding. I was so upset that this had happened, especially when it was referred to by my GP as "a threatened miscarriage". I began to fear not *whether* I would lose the baby, but *when*. Of course I blamed myself: the way I walked, the way I got up from chairs, and so many other things I did, all of which put extra strain on my stomach. I can also remember thinking that people wouldn't be at all surprised if I lost the baby, almost as though they were expecting it to happen, and I hated that thought. I wanted so much to achieve this, to carry this baby to term, to be a mother and responsible for another life. And to show people that it is possible to care for a baby in ways other than the conventional ways that are taken for granted.

I was aware that I would really be breaking new ground in

finding alternative ways of caring for the child. I hoped that my experiences would give encouragement to other disabled mothers, especially the ones that didn't have the use of their arms.

It was decided that I should go into hospital for a short time on bed rest, in the hope that the bleeding might stop. There was also the suggestion that I might be having twins! That really would be a challenge for me now, wouldn't it? I can remember lying in bed in the Brighton General Hospital almost too frightened to move, in case I should lose my baby. For a few days I didn't get out of bed at all, not even to go to the toilet.

There was an irony to those few days of my life. A young girl in the bed next to mine told me that she had come into hospital hoping to have an abortion. She was in her teens, and spoke of her pregnancy with great irritation, saying it was a mistake. From the subsequent conversation she had with the doctor, it seemed that this was not her first unwanted pregnancy, and her request was refused. She was furious about this, and began weeping and wailing about her life being ruined. As I watched her pack her bag and walk out of the ward still carrying her baby, albeit begrudgingly, I prayed that I could keep mine.

Gradually, the bleeding stopped and I was allowed out of bed to walk to the bathroom. I used to break out in a cold sweat, hardly daring to move at first, dreading that awful feeling of losing blood. But thankfully it didn't happen again, and after ten days I went home.

The antenatal clinic was the first place I became aware of the patronising way I would be treated by some people with regard to my pregnancy. Ken had time off work to help me at these appointments, and the nurses would often talk to him rather than to me. They would ask him questions about me such as "Can she manage to undress herself?"and "Can she manage to give us a specimen of urine?"

I found this attitude amazing, especially as these people were nurses. They must have thought me to be deaf, stupid and incapable of understanding language, and what was more ridiculous was that when they did speak to me, they raised their voices to almost shouting level. On one occasion I asked a nurse whether she had heard of polio, whether she knew what it was. While she gaped at me, I informed her that although my limbs were affected, my brain was fully intact. Then it was her turn to be amazed! I do not suffer fools gladly, and quickly put them straight on the fact that I can answer for myself.

My obstetrician, Mr Bostock, who looked a bit like Neil Diamond, was never patronising. He had a great sense of humour, and from the outset said he didn't doubt that I would find ways in which to care for my baby. This gave me great encouragement, of which I was in real need by that time. He discussed with me the chances of my delivery being normal, and he felt that if possible we should avoid a caesarean section—mainly, he said, because afterwards my stomach would be very painful and prohibit me from being able to sit up or move around for a few days. Knowing how much I wanted to care for my baby, I would find this very frustrating, so he had decided to opt for a normal delivery.

Jill Rockey was the other person who was very positive about my abilities, and together we discussed possible ways of dressing the baby. From sewing buttons and elastic loops on to nappies and strips of velcro onto garments, replacing buttons and making a sling for me to carry the baby in, there was no-one who encouraged me more than Jill. Having spent her working life around disabled people, she knew so much was possible. Although she had no children herself, she knew me well, and her dealings with disabled people had taught her that nothing is impossible if you really want to achieve it.

I had already decided that I would not breast feed the baby. Although on the face of it this option seems easier, there being no bottles to hold and no feeds to prepare, it would mean that I would have to keep getting partially undressed throughout the day, and this would be very tiring for me.

Towards the latter part of my pregnancy, I was visited by an elderly lady who introduced herself as my health visitor. Her name was Miss Roberts, and from the expression on her face when we first met she was obviously quite unprepared for the degree of my disability. She proceeded to ask me all the questions she could think of about how I would care for my baby. My answers were very positive; there was no room for doubt or negativity when speaking to these professionals. They were, I knew, in very powerful positions and if they felt that I was not capable of looking after the baby, my greatest fear—that I wouldn't be able to keep it—might be realised.

I explained that she must appreciate how new all this was to me, but that it was my intention to deal with each problem as I came to it; and although I felt very much under pressure to convince her that I was capable of looking after this child, in her defence I must say that I found her quite pleasant. She was not a mother herself, which was rather disconcerting as obviously she had no first-hand personal experience. Her first visit ended with her suggestion to me that perhaps it would be best if, while I was alone with the baby, I didn't attempt to do anything with it that involved using water. She was obviously terrified that I would drown it!

For the remaining months of my pregnancy, I walked as little as possible to avoid falling. My balance, though never good, was even more precarious, and getting up from the sitting position was an adventure in itself!

The delivery date was September 11th, though by mid-

August I could hardly keep my balance at all. Mr Bostock had suggested that if the baby was not born before the end of August, I should be admitted to hospital and the birth induced, because of the difficulty I was having with walking and generally moving about. So on the August Bank Holiday Monday of 1978, I went into hospital.

I had particularly asked to be in a room on my own because I knew that it would take time and lots of trial and error before I worked out how I would cope with the various tasks of caring for my baby. The last thing I wanted was to be stared at whilst I experimented; this was something I would have to be left alone to deal with. I was under enough pressure as it was, although determined to succeed, and I certainly didn't want to be on show at what I felt was a private time.

On the following morning, Tuesday 30th August at about 11 o'clock, they began inducing the birth, and a doctor began probing around inside me, with what looked like a crochet hook, to break my waters. I had now been put into one of the delivery rooms; it was very sparse and as well as my bed, there was only a cot in the corner. As my labour proceeded, I envisaged my son or daughter lying in this, which was very encouraging.

Beside all my feelings of anticipation of this great event, I was so excited and just couldn't wait to see this baby, to finally hold it and to be a mother. Ken was sitting beside me, and as the hours went by and nothing much was happening, we both began to be concerned. The pain had become stronger each time the nurse came in and turned the switch on the drip that had been inserted into my hand to increase the strength of the contractions, and she said it would become more painful as time went on.

I was being checked regularly to see how dilated my cervix was becoming, but things were not moving along as quickly as had been hoped. By late afternoon I was very tired and in a great deal of pain, and despite the prior misgivings my obstetrician had mentioned about me having a caesarian section, this was now being considered as a possibility.

A further complication was having the drip inserted into my hand rather than my arm. This was necessary because my arms are very thin due to the paralysis, making it almost impossible to find a vein in which to insert a needle. However, my hand was becoming bruised and I was getting very tired.

It was late evening when I was taken to the operating theatre. I was by now drifting in and out of consciousness and the pain was excruciating. I was not able to push hard enough because my tummy muscles were so weak. The theatre sister made some sort of a splint and strapped my hand to it to prevent it from slipping down and the needle coming out. It was discussed whether I might benefit from an epidural, but after a phone call to Mr Bostock, it became apparent that this was not an option: the curvature of my spine would make an epidural dangerous.

Each time I became conscious, Ken was there looking worried and not knowing what he could do to help. He was giving me pain-relieving gas and air. Normally this works by putting a gas mask over your face as soon as you feel a contraction. However, if you're not able to do it yourself, you have to yell out each time you get a pain, and the person helping you must be very immediate with the mask in order for it to help you. Consequently this pain relief was a bit hit and miss!

It was eventually decided that forceps should be used to help delivery. By now it was after 3 o'clock in the morning, and a doctor was called from his bed to perform this task. I can remember seeing his blonde head over the huge lump of my stomach as he put his hand inside me to feel where the baby's eyes were so as not to harm them with the forceps. This was extremely painful and I screamed out.

"Do you want this baby or not?" he asked me in a very irate voice (men!).

"Of course I do!" I yelled at him. "What do you think I've been doing for the past day?"

His reply was to order me to push as hard as I could on the next contraction, which I duly did, and at 3.30 am on August 31, 1978 my darling Emma Lynne was born. The nurse laid Emma on my chest; she was so beautiful and her skin was like that of a peach. She wasn't covered in blood and mess as I had expected; there was a little bit in her hair, but apart from that she looked so lovely, with dark hair and big blue eyes.

Ken was crying beside me, it was so hard to take in this wonderful event, this beautiful baby that was ours. She weighed 6lb 9oz, and after an examination the doctor told us that she was in perfect health. I was so tired and so relieved to be free of the pain, which had seemed to have lasted a lifetime. But when I looked at my wonderful daughter Emma, it had been worth every second of pain to have brought her into the world.

After a few hours of well earned rest, I awoke back in my room with Emma in her cot beside my bed. Although I was feeling quite sore after giving birth, I managed to sit up in bed and asked the nurse to lift Emma on to my lap. I must admit to feeling very nervous now that the baby was born and needing care. I gently manoeuvred her little body between my knees, lifting her head with my hand and resting it on my left knee, putting my leg around her to cradle her. She seemed quite happy nestling there.

"That's how I'll cuddle you, little Emma," I told her, and then, keeping her in this position and holding her feeding bottle in my right hand, I gave Emma her first feed. When it came to bringing up Emma's wind I sat her up and very gently rocked her back and forth, which to my great relief resulted in a burp!

Over the next few days in hospital, my confidence in caring for Emma began to grow. I quickly discarded the sling that had been made for me to carry her in, as she seemed to get lost in it and didn't feel close enough to me, and I lifted her by holding the front of her clothes in my teeth. After a little trial and error I found that the all-in-one garments known as 'babygrows' were the ideal clothes for lifting her, as her body remained straight in these.

The nursing staff were excellent, and left me to get on with it just as I had asked, and should I have needed any help I only had to ring the bell. The first time that I fed Emma, winded her and lifted her back into her cot where she snuggled down to sleep, I felt absolutely elated! It made me feel really powerful and useful, feelings that I hadn't often experienced. The nurses were bathing her, as I had not crossed that bridge yet, but gradually I was able to dress her myself, though getting those tiny arms into sleeves, and legs into leg holes was not easy.

Fastening the poppers with my teeth took a while to perfect, because I couldn't actually see which bit fitted where, but had to feel with my tongue. As with everything else, however, it became easier with practice. My parents came to see their first grandchild while I was in hospital; they were delighted with her and with how I was managing to look after her, and their faces glowed with pride.

When I left hospital, Ken stayed at home with us for two weeks, during which time I continued learning how to care for my baby. I have never been so tired in my life. I worried about the length of time it took me to do some things such as dressing Emma. This could take up to an hour, and it also required a great deal of effort on both our parts, as we had to be very patient. There was no point in Ken doing it, as he would soon be returning to work—and anyway, I wanted to do it. Ken prepared all the day's feeds the night before; it was one task I was not able to do, because the bottles obviously had to be done up tightly as well as shaken vigorously to mix the feed properly.

I was very apprehensive the first morning that Emma and I were left alone. Yes, I knew I could manage to do most of the things I had to by now, but it's different if you know there's someone around in case things don't go quite as planned: then you have fewer worries should something awful occur. Now I was on my own and the baby was totally dependent on me.

eight

THE first few days that I was on my own with Emma were, to say the least, very nerve-wracking for me. I remember feeling very alone with this tiny, helpless baby and the mammoth task of looking after her, although at the same time I knew that was the way it had to be. It would be impossible for me to have an able-bodied person around, as they would, naturally enough, want to help me; and I knew that any such 'help' would result in them taking over. And that definitely wasn't going to happen—Emma was *my* baby.

Despite wanting to desperately, which lead to me arguing with myself as to whether or not I could manage this alone, I didn't actually bath Emma during the day, but would wait until Ken came home to help. Instead, each morning I would get a small tub of water and just wash her face and bottom.

However, after a few weeks my confidence grew. I knew she would feel better for having a soak, so I came up with a scheme: I lifted her carry cot out of its frame and put the baby bath in it, then I wheeled it into the bathroom and put a few jugs of water in it, just enough to cover Emma's bottom. I then wheeled the bath back into the bedroom where Emma was lying on the double bed. After undressing her, I lined her up with the bath, which was positioned at the bottom of the bed, and slid her

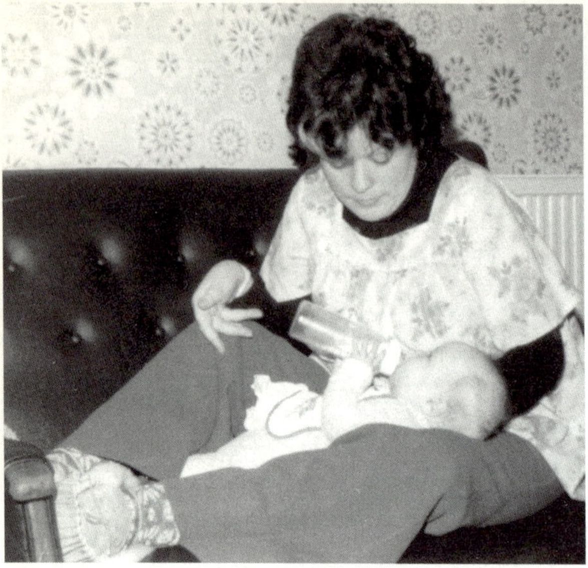

Feeding Emma, back home, 1979

down into the water by holding her legs.

I make no bones about it, the first few times I did this I was really nervous, but after a while we both became more relaxed and Emma began to giggle as I made a game of sliding her into the bath. She enjoyed it, and so did I.

Getting Emma *out* of the bath, though, was not quite so straightforward. After much trial and error this was accomplished by gently pulling her arm until most of her body was on the towel which I had laid out on the bed, then it was a question of rolling her in the towel onto the bed. She would often fall asleep while I dried and dressed her (as did I occasionally, such was the effort on my part).

My reward, however, was seeing her clean and comfortable in her pram. I had given up with the terry towelling nappies with buttons and loops; they were too large and kept slipping off. I began using disposable ones with sticky tapes on each side, which were a very new invention in those days. I would spread the nappy out, and gently pull Emma on to it by holding her ankles in my fingers, then undo the sticky tape before pulling the centre of the nappy up between Emma's legs. Whilst holding the centre of the nappy with my hand, I would pull the tape over in my lips and press it down with my chin. In those days, if you didn't get a tape in the right place at the first attempt, it would lose its adhesive and not stick a second time, which was very frustrating for us both.

I began to notice over the next few months that Ken was not very patient with Emma, especially when she cried a lot. Emma would not seem very relaxed when her father held her and this worried me, as I wondered whether the contrast between how I handled Emma and how her father did was confusing to her. Whatever the reason, it made Ken irritable, as he was not a confident person anyway. Caring for a baby the first time round is unknown ground for every parent, so I just put it down to the fact that Ken was nervous about holding the baby.

As well as the day-to-day care of Emma, there was also the question of taking her out. Obviously I couldn't walk along pushing her pram, and the only form of mobility I had was my three-wheeler invalid carriage—in which I could take no passengers. So when we did our weekly shop on Saturdays Emma would be strapped to Ken in a baby harness and they would go on the bus, while I drove my car to Sainsbury's and met them there. Then once Ken had got my wheelchair out of my car, he would sit Emma on my lap and push us both round the supermarket with one hand, and handle the trolley with the other.

This was obviously a very difficult situation. Ken would get very short-tempered, which Emma would pick up on and cry, making her father more irritated. I hated these times, as I felt out of control of the situation. After a few months of this, we decided to get a baby-sitter to stay with Emma while we did the shopping.

On one particular occasion Ken's short temper got the better of him. It happened when Emma was about eight months old and teething. She had been crying on and off for most of the day and there had been no way of comforting her. She was hot and obviously in a lot of pain from her gums. I had been rubbing her gums with gel, which gave her some relief but not for very long.

It was a testing situation, but I didn't realise how hard it was for Ken to keep his cool. He had gone into the bedroom to see to Emma, and suddenly the tone of her crying changed. I knew something was wrong and walked into the bedroom. I simply couldn't believe my eyes: Ken, with a look of fury on his face, was holding Emma and shaking her. Her head was rocking back and forth, and I screamed at him to put her down.

As well as being completely horrified by what I saw, I was frustrated by my inability to do anything physically. I wanted to grab her away from him—this was my precious child, my baby. He had completely lost control of himself and could well have given her brain damage. After the event he was pitifully sorry, but I found this as hard to deal with as his lack of patience.

This was not an easy time for us, and it wasn't helped by the fact that I was unable to take Emma out of the flat independently. I often had the feeling that the two of us were imprisoned there, and found it very oppressive.

What I really wanted was a proper car in which I could drive my family. Ken had never driven and wasn't very keen to learn, although this seemed to most people to be the obvious answer. I contacted our local MP at the time, Andrew Bowden, who visited us promptly. He was a pleasant man of about fifty, and showed great concern for our situation. I asked him about the question of the government providing me with a vehicle more suitable to the needs of us as a family.

It was at this time that the government began phasing out the invalid three-wheelers. There had been many complaints about these cars: as well as the fact that no passengers could be taken in them, they were not very safe and were unstable in the wind. So it was that an organisation called Motability came into being. It was government-backed and was intended to provide disabled drivers with vehicles which they could have for three years on a leasing scheme, paid for with their mobility benefit. At the end of the three years the car would be returned and put up for auction; the disabled person then got another car for another three years, and so on.

This scheme was fine for those disabled people who didn't need a great deal of modification done to a vehicle to enable them to drive it. For instance, if you only needed a steering knob, or a minor alteration done that could easily be removed, or if you were a disabled passenger and wished to remain so, you would reap the benefits of the scheme. But for others like myself who needed a heavily adapted vehicle, it wasn't really cost effective to remove what would be quite expensive facilities such as foot steering, costing over £1000, after only three years.

So what I wanted Mr Bowden to do was to try and initiate a different type of scheme, whereby the disabled person could buy the vehicle from Motability using their mobility allowance, and make use of the vehicle in the long term. The Minister for the Disabled at the time was Alf Morris, and Andrew Bowden wrote to him on our behalf. After a few weeks he came back to us, saying that it had been decided to hold an Adjournment Debate on our situation. This meant basically that at the end of the day's business in the House of Commons, a Member of Parliament could discuss the problems of a particular constituent in the House with the Minister in charge of the relevant Department.

Ken and I were invited to attend, which we did, taking Emma

with us. She was then about eight months old and she liked laying on her tummy in her carry cot, lifting her head up to peer out. I will always treasure the memory of her, having been set down near a statue of Sir Winston Churchill by a helpful policeman, lifting her head up and gazing over the side and giving a huge dribbly grin as if to say, "What am I doing here, Mum?"!

The debate lasted for some 20 minutes, after which we were introduced to Alf Morris, who said he would do all he could to help. Because the case had been taken up by our MP, we had some publicity both in the local press and a couple of women's magazines, in one of which I was called 'Mother Courage', a title which I have never quite lived down!

Eventually Motability brought in a second scheme permitting people to buy their vehicles, and I became the proud owner of a Mini Clubman Estate, which had foot steering put in by a gentleman called David Hodge. David was second to none in these matters; he was a great motorbike enthusiast and an excellent mechanic, and it is because of his foresight and efforts that I and many other disabled people have had the opportunity of driving. I am eternally indebted to him; nothing was too much trouble for David, and if something wouldn't work out one way then he'd try another and another until he succeeded in helping me attain my goal—to drive, and take my family out with me. One of his sayings I remember was, "A little help is worth a lot of pity." He has long since retired, but his grandson (also called David) has inherited his brilliance. He has taken over the business and continues to enable disabled people to have great independence.

The vehicle was left hand drive, because I had to steer with my right foot and because of the positioning of the accelerator and brake, but wasn't too much of a problem apart from when I needed to overtake another vehicle.

Although I had been driving my three-wheeler for some time, I still had to have driving lessons in my new car, and quite rightly had to pass the same test as everyone else, the only concession being that I was permitted an extra twenty minutes in which to complete it.

I really enjoyed driving my car and wished my lessons could go on and on, though I must admit I did find the steering very heavy. It was not possible to have power assisted steering, as the Mini was too small to incorporate it under the bonnet. I failed my first driving test, in Hove, for cutting a corner and, although I was desperately disappointed there was nothing for it but to do it again as soon as possible.

My second was taken in Eastbourne, and I was delighted at the end when the examiner told me I had passed. I remember that day in 1980 so well, and when I drove Emma to the park on my own, I felt as though everyone knew I had just passed my test and was watching me!

Emma was really excited about going out in my car. It was a two door, so she had to learn to climb into her little seat, which was behind mine. Because I knew I wouldn't be able to reach to fasten the security buckle, I contacted my friends at Chailey Heritage for advice. They told me about a child's car seat, which was like a table that fitted round the child and could be adjusted from the driver's seat on the same fitting as the front seat belt. This meant I could tighten the table around Emma once she had got herself into it, which she did with lots of verbal encouragement from me and, on days she was not feeling so co-operative, the bribery of sweets! Once Emma was sitting down, I could tighten the tray around her by pulling the strap with my teeth, and release it in the same way. While this was still a novelty Emma always co-operated, but sometimes if she was tired or didn't want to be bothered it made life a bit difficult. Basically I relied on her help, and usually I was able to talk her into her seat.

I expressed my concern to the council about us being in the flat with the balcony once Emma had begun getting around on her own. Toddlers are renowned for getting themselves into trouble, sometimes with horrifying results. The thought of Emma falling over the balcony entered my head regularly once she could move more quickly than I could. Should so dreadful a thing have happened there would undoubtedly have been people who said, "I don't expect the mother could cope with the child."

I had no intention, however, of waiting until it did, and spoke frequently on the phone to Brighton Council about this. It so happened that a new block of flats was being built just down the road from where we were living. After being told that there was no chance of us having a bungalow—which was what we really needed—I asked whether we could be considered for a ground floor flat.

We had to wait a few months before we were moved. The flats were specifically built for the elderly, so were by no means perfect. There was no garden or safe enclosed area where Emma could play, as I had so hoped there would be. In those days housing for disabled people was practically non-existent. The council had recently built a few bungalows specifically for this purpose, but they were in an area notorious for its social problems called the Whitehawk Estate.

Vandalism and burglary were rife there, and unruly youths made the lives of some of the residents of the estate an absolute misery. Disabled people were a particular target for these youths, so that, despite being housed in a property which met the needs of their disabilities, these people often had no peace in their homes. Stones were thrown at them over their garden walls, and they were called names such as 'spastic', the word applied to anyone with any disability at that time by ignorant people.

Our flat was situated on the edge of the estate, and happily we were not pestered by troublemakers. Underneath the flat was the car park, which had a steep bank down to it along with a path, but I didn't use it to park my car as I couldn't have coped with the walk.

We had not been in our new home for very long before, on the way out one day, Emma decided she would run down the bank to see the cars. Although I was really frightened that she would get hurt, I knew that the more I shouted at her to come back the more she would not. She was testing me, to see how much she could get away with, knowing that I couldn't run after her. I just got into my car which was parked outside the front of our flat, and started to drive away. As I had hoped, this brought my daughter running up the bank screaming and crying at the thought of me leaving her, and after a good telling off, she never did it again.

I had of course been totally helpless in that situation. Emma's mobility outdid mine, though I always thought it very important not to stress that point to her; she could see it for herself, and I never wanted her to use it against me. Especially if I was trying to get her to do something that she didn't want to do.

At this time in our lives, Emma and I were socially very isolated. As I wasn't living near my family I only saw them when I drove up to Ashford about once a month, or now and then when they visited me. My father's car breaking business took up most of his time, and he never was a great one for visiting, because he didn't enjoy driving much. As so often happens when you don't live close to people, they are wrapped up in their world and you get on with yours. I was very lonely for adult company, and apart from Ken who was at work all day, I had no-one to talk to of my age.

Fortunately, though, I then made contact with a lady called June. I had placed an advert in the doctor's surgery for someone to help me bath Emma in the mornings and June had answered it. Although I would have loved to be able to continue bathing Emma independently, once she was about 9 months old she was too heavy and I could no longer bath her in the same way I had when she was tiny. So June would come in before she went to work at the hospital where she was a nurse. She was in her mid forties and had two children, and she had recently lost her husband through cancer.

June became a good friend, and as I got to know her better I found that I could confide in her. I told her that there were difficulties with Ken and Emma and that after I had seen him shaking her, things began to change between us. I never forgave him, although when things were going well between us, I told myself that I did. It was good to be able to be honest with someone about our troubles, and to be able to tell someone that this was one reason that I looked for private help with bathing Emma.

June was the only person I told about Ken; I didn't want anyone else to know anything about this. I was so disappointed with him; physically it was so much easier for him to do things for her than it was for me, but he just couldn't cope emotionally. I didn't understand why he was always on such a short fuse with Emma. At that time he wouldn't really talk about his problem, but I did suggest he get some help, or just go and talk his feelings out with someone. But he wasn't interested then, and looking back, although it was hard to witness his tempers, it was almost as bad to see his remorse afterwards, which I'm afraid cut no ice with me.

nine

By the time she was eighteen months old, Emma was seriously in need of other children to mix with. One day I saw a notice in the library about a mother and toddler group which was being set up. I had not mixed socially for so long that I knew it would be difficult for me to mix with people again, but I also knew it would do both Emma and I good to get out of the flat and to interact with other people.

On the first day that we went along to the group I felt very self-conscious of my disability, my main worry being, as always, that I didn't fall over. However, children always give plenty of opportunities for conversation to flow and are good ice breakers. They asked me the usual questions, to the horror of their embarrassed mothers.

"Why do you walk funny?" and "What's the matter with your leg?" are the two I remember most, and I answered with as much honesty as I could, saying that when I was a little girl I had been very ill. This usually satisfied their natural inquisitiveness; children that age have none of the inhibitions of adults, and they accepted the straightforward explanation.

Emma didn't understand what they were talking about; after all, I was perfectly normal to her. She loved playing with the other children, however, and made friends quickly. There were about six other mothers in the group, some of whom already knew one another. Although I was aware of the predictable awkwardness on both my part and that of the other mothers on the first few occasions that we met up, it soon disappeared once we began talking, and I felt really good about taking part.

Although I got on well with the other mums, I made a special friend of a German girl called Benita. She was really friendly, and before very long Benita and I would meet up regularly and go to the nearby park with the children, chatting while they played. Benita's son Ben was the same age as Emma, and they too became firm friends. I loved watching Emma run around and enjoy herself. She was such a good child, although very strong willed!

I put Emma's name down for playschool, which she could attend when she was three. It was close by, and I didn't think that she would have a problem parting from me as she was quite a confident child. However, on the morning that I took her to meet her teacher and see where she would be going, things turned out differently than I expected. There was a step up into the building which I couldn't manage, and because of this I told Emma to go in and find the teacher and bring her to Mummy. Emma began to cry, saying that she didn't want to go in because Mummy couldn't, and try as I might, I couldn't persuade her otherwise. I called out, and eventually got the teacher's attention. She was a lady in her early fifties, and came over straight away. I explained about my disability and that Emma wasn't happy to go in without me.

"Oh, don't worry about that, Emma," she said. "We have another door that doesn't have a step. Shall we let Mummy in that one?" At this suggestion the tears stopped, Emma nodded and a smile spread across her face. Once I was inside and sitting down, Emma went off with the teacher to meet the other children and soon she was playing happily.

When the day came for her to go to playschool for real, she went in quite happily with the teacher, who met her from my car. Although the door without the step wasn't used very often, Emma would always point to it when we arrived at playschool and say "Mummy's door"!

By the time Emma was two, she could virtually dress herself, with my verbal guidance. The main things we found very frustrating were putting her socks on; she could do it, but often they were on back to front! When I tried to help her with them one morning by getting them on her the right way around, I accidentally bit her toe! She screamed at me, and I felt dreadful! The other thing that took us ages was fastening buttons. Emma's little fingers couldn't do it, and my fingers just wouldn't grip the buttons. After we'd both struggled, we often used to end up giggling, and would congratulate each other as, with perseverance, things were achieved!

Emma soon settled into playschool, although she did have a bit of trouble with at first with her drawings, which she would do by holding the pencil in her mouth, like Mummy! It took a while to get her to use her hand, but eventually she did and found it much easier.

Early in 1982 I discovered that I was expecting another baby. We were delighted with the news, as were our families. I felt really sick during the first couple of months of this pregnancy, far worse than when I had been pregnant with Emma. We were offered a council house now, and I was so pleased that Emma would be able to play in the garden at last. She was three and a half and was very excited about having a brother or sister, and every day she would ask me how long it would be before the baby came.

Our new home had three bedrooms, and a stairlift was installed by the council to enable me to get upstairs. As the previous tenant was also disabled, a bathroom with a shower and toilet had been built downstairs. The garden was a bit of a disappointment for me, because it had some steps leading up to it, but Emma thought it was marvellous to have so much space to play in.

When I was four months pregnant, I lost a lot of blood, more than I had when expecting Emma, which had been bad enough. We called the doctor, who said that all I could do was to go to bed and stay there for at least a week, in the hope that things would settle down. That week was one of the longest in my life. As before, I hardly dared move in case I lost this baby. Ken had time off work to help with Emma and look after me. For the most part, things had improved somewhat between Ken and Emma as she got older, and only became heated when Ken would ask her to do something she didn't want to do. She was, as I have said, very strong-willed and would often court confrontation with her father.

When the doctor returned at the end of the week and put a machine on my stomach to listen for the baby's heartbeat, thankfully it was loud and clear. The bleeding had almost stopped, so I was allowed to get up, though obviously I had to be very careful about moving around too much. By now Emma was going to playschool every morning, and as soon as the bleeding stopped I was glad to be able to resume taking her in the car. She would start full time at school in September of that year, when she would be four. The new baby was due on 1st October, so I would be able to give it plenty of attention, and having already succeeded with caring for Emma, I wasn't worried about things so much this time round.

It was the beginning of the last week in June, and I still had three months of my pregnancy to go. We had just finished lunch one Saturday, and Ken was clearing away the dishes. I had just sat down on the toilet when the most amazing thing happened. I felt something, which at the time to my horror, I thought was my baby's head, outside my body. I could feel this thing moving around beneath me as I sat on the toilet. Hardly daring to breathe for fear of what might happen next, I called Ken. When he looked down, he said there was something long hanging out of me and it was moving around, and that whatever it was, it certainly did not look like a baby's head. I sat rigidly still and told him to ring for an ambulance; whatever it was that was coming away from me I could not imagine.

When the paramedics arrived, they told me that what had come outside my body was in fact one of the baby's legs in the foetal sack. By this time, I was absolutely terrified and in a cold sweat; I didn't want to move in case the baby came out completely and fell into the toilet, but the paramedic insisted I get on to the ambulance chair. I managed to do this, though laying on it rather than sitting, for obvious reasons.

Emma was crying, obviously having no understanding what was going on, and Ken asked the neighbour next door to look after her while we went to the hospital. Once inside the ambulance I was laid down, pillows were placed under my lower back and my bottom raised in order to encourage the baby's leg back inside me. When we arrived at the hospital, I was immediately put on a drip to delay contractions, and the baby's heartbeat closely monitored. Fortunately the heartbeat was still strong, but I was told that as the foetal sack had ruptured, the main danger now was infection entering it.

I was by this time 25 weeks pregnant, much too early for the baby to be born, and it was decided that I should spend the remainder of my pregnancy in hospital on bed rest. The thought of three months in hospital was really depressing, and what about Emma? Ken had to go to work—how would he be able to cope? However, once I thought about it, I realised that I could do nothing but comply; this baby was also important and we owed it the very best chance of being born healthy. I questioned the hospital staff about the possibility of the baby being alive if it was born this soon; they spoke as though there really wasn't much likelihood of it surviving, saying that at this stage of its development, its lungs were still very immature. Basically it just wasn't ready to be born yet.

I spent the next three days sitting in bed reading and worrying about what was going to happen. The thought of all those weeks until October stretching before me seemed like an eternity. Ken was off work for the time being, and brought Emma to see me every day after her morning at school. I hoped and prayed that she would be good for him.

On the Wednesday afternoon I began having pains in my stomach, which I recognised as labour pains, despite the fact that I was being given a drug intravenously to prevent labour starting. I told the nurse who was looking after me, and she said it was more likely to be constipation. As the evening wore on I knew quite well it wasn't constipation; I'd had this pain before, and by midnight I was in agony. I had been told, on admission to the hospital, that should I need an emergency delivery it would have to be by caesarian section, as it was thought that there was no way the baby would survive a natural birth.

At about 1.00 am I called the nurse, saying that my baby was coming, and she bought me a bedpan! I couldn't help but bear down, and as I did so, blood shot across the room, hitting the opposite wall. Then, all hell broke loose as the bedpan was snatched away and my bed was wheeled across the corridor to the operating theatre. Medical staff were rushing in all directions, shouting instructions to each other. I was feeling frantic.

"Please don't let my baby die," I prayed over and over, crossing my legs firmly and screaming that it was too soon. Almost as soon as my bed had been pushed through the double doors of the theatre, and I was about to be given an injection in preparation for a caesarian, I felt the baby coming.

Suddenly everything was quiet, almost surreal, as I watched this tiny baby slip easily out of my body. Then I felt numb and could only stare down at what I had given birth to, feeling both shock and disbelief at once. Yes, it had two arms and two legs, a head, even fingers and toes, but it was so tiny, so unbelievably tiny, that my eyes could not take in what they were seeing. I didn't know whether it was male or female at that point in time, because it looked so unfinished; the little bubble of skin it had between its legs could have been either. The skin was transparent like tissue paper; I could see veins through it, the ears had no substance to them, and were rolled up close to a head that couldn't have been any bigger than a tennis ball. The eyes were not yet ready to open, but I could see movement beneath the lids. The baby opened its mouth, took a gasp and let out a cry that sounded as though it had come from a million miles away. As it did so, its whole body contorted with the effort of desperately trying to breathe.

I continued to gaze entranced at this absurdly small scrap of humanity that was my child, as the nursing staff carried on around me, doing what needed to be done.

"Well done Maureen," said the Sister, "you have a little girl."

"Have I?" I answered. I felt neither happy or sad at that point, only bewildered. As soon as the cord was cut, the baby was wrapped up and I was told that they were taking her up to the Special Care Baby Unit situated on the floor above. They said I could go up and see her once she had been attended to and I had been cleaned up. Although everything seemed unreal, I kept trying to explain to myself what had happened, trying to get it into my head so that I actually believed it, but I couldn't.

"Will she die?" I asked.

"They'll do all they can for her upstairs," was the Sister's reply.

An hour or so later, I was helped into a wheelchair and a porter took me upstairs in the lift, the night's events slowly beginning to penetrate my mind. I felt so alone amid this enormous turn of events. The birth had been so completely different from Emma's; there had been no pain, no stitches or forceps, just a slight sensation of pushing something out of me, and then it had all been over.

It was almost two o'clock in the morning when I was pushed into the Special Care Baby Unit by a nurse who was waiting for me. The unit was divided into cubicles with about four incubators in each, containing tiny babies being kept alive by so many wires and monitors that their tiny bodies were barely visible. I had entered into a world that I had never imagined existed, a world which, at the time, I would rather never have had cause to enter. Monitors clicked resolutely, their screens displaying the vital information about each baby as it clung to life in its artificial shell, rather than its mother's womb, where nature had intended it still to be growing and nourished.

When we reached the incubator that held my daughter, I saw that she had been attached to a monitor, which clicked at her every breath. She had a tube in her mouth attached to a ventilator that was breathing for her, her lungs being too immature to manage this independently. She had a pink doll's hat on to help keep her warm, and her arms and legs, which were about the thickness of a woman's finger, were moving about. I asked whether the baby was in pain; the nurse replied that although she wasn't, she was a very small baby even by the unit's standards, and that at the moment things must be taken hour by hour. She said that I should be prepared for anything, that the baby's birth weight was just 1lb 13oz and she would lose weight before she gained any. The phrase 'less than a bag of sugar' came to me then. It seemed impossible she could be so very premature and still be alive.

I was asked whether I would like my daughter christened, there being no guarantees that she would live for very long. I agreed to this and asked the nurse to ring Ken, who was still blissfully unaware of the events of the night. As I sat beside my daughter, gazing sometimes into the black inky darkness outside the windows, tears which had up until now been blocked by the shock of all that had happened made their way down my cheeks, and sobs shook my body. I faced the very real possibility that my baby would die, that I may never know her, touch her, see her smile and grow up, and I wished desperately that I could have kept her inside me for long enough.

When the nurse returned she comforted me, saying there was a chance, though small, that my child would survive. She said that these babies really put up a fight for their lives, and for some reason it was more often the girls than the boys that won the fight. The priest was on his way, so as she was going to be christened I had to give my daughter a name. I decided to call her Lucy Rose as I'd always liked the name Lucy, and the rose is my favourite flower. It had not been possible to contact Ken, he was probably fast asleep and I didn't want the nurse to keep on ringing in case she woke Emma, who would be frightened in the dark.

When the priest arrived, it was with great relief that I recognised him to be someone I knew from my school days, who had often visited Chailey. His name was Father Gerald Coates, and he had also christened Emma, albeit in much happier circumstances. He was of great comfort to me that night of 30th June 1982, as in the early hours of the morning, with the nurse completing our small congregation he christened Lucy Rose and prayed for her to live. After the very moving little service I went back to my room, and Father Gerald sat with me until I fell asleep, totally exhausted from the traumas I had been through.

When I awoke in the morning, the first words that I said were, "Is Lucy still alive?" When I was told that she was, I just wanted to be with her. After breakfast I was taken up to the baby unit where I remained for the rest of the morning. Ken had by now been contacted and he arrived after dropping Emma at school. He was staggered at the sight of his daughter and at the events of the previous night, and was more than a little apologetic that he hadn't heard the phone. The nursing staff on the unit were second to none in their care of Lucy, but reminded us constantly that although she was doing very well, we had to take things hour by hour for the immediate future. Premature babies as small as Lucy were extremely unpredictable, and one major danger to them was the risk of infection which they were totally unable to fight, due to their immune system not being mature. So we had to wear hospital gowns which were sterile when we were in the unit and wash our hands regularly.

Lucy continued to do well, and at the end of each day I would tell her how many days she had lived, how much we all loved her, and about her big sister Emma who was longing to hold her. Emma did get a glimpse of her baby sister during those early days of Lucy's life, but she was quite concerned at all the wires and equipment that surrounded the tiny infant. Because Lucy didn't look like the babies Emma had seen, she wasn't very impressed with her sister!

As she entered her second week, Lucy was being taken off the ventilator for a few hours a day and breathing for herself. This was a really big landmark; the sooner premature babies can do this, the greater chance they have of life, as it helps the lungs to mature. The effort this took Lucy was clearly visible by the way her tiny rib cage distended each time she drew breath in, and she soon became tired. We were now allowed to open the port holes in the side of the incubator and put our hands in to touch Lucy.

This proved difficult for me as I am not able to lift my arm, so the nurse opened one side of the incubator and slid Lucy out slightly, which enabled me to reach her. At first this was only possible for a minute or two, as Lucy's body temperature dropped very quickly. All the time the incubator was open, Lucy had oxygen held under her nose. As she was not able to suck at this stage, Lucy was fed intravenously by a tube that went into her stomach through her nose. She was fed my milk, which I expressed daily through a pump. I felt like a cow being milked when using it, but I wanted to give Lucy every chance and believed that mother's milk is the best for a baby as tiny as Lucy was.

At this stage, we were allowed to start taking part in Lucy's daily care. This involved cleaning her mouth, which became very dry as there was no fluid going into it. It was done twice daily with a wet cotton bud which, incredibly, almost filled her mouth up. We could also wash her face and bottom, being very careful not to get water on any other part of her body, as this would affect her body temperature and she would become too cold. She would not be able to have a bath until she weighed one kilo, we were told, but it was great to be able to do these

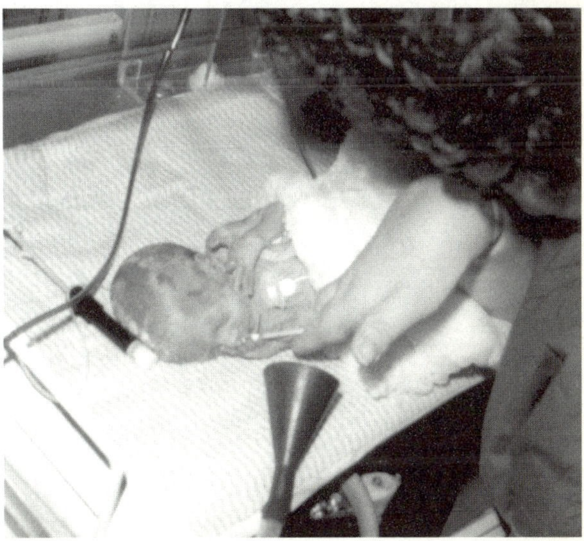

Lucy in hospital incubator

small things for Lucy. It made more real to me the fact that I had just given birth; it had been very hard not being able to hold her when she had been born, and having her snatched away immediately.

By now, Lucy's eyes had begun to open and specks of blue were visible through tiny gaps beneath her eyelids. She continued to wear the doll's hat all the time to keep her head warm, and her nappies were cut down from normal size new-born babies' nappies, as these would have been enormous on her. Actually they were so unbelievably tiny that I really wish I had kept one, though at the time I didn't want any souvenirs; getting through each day was enough to cope with.

I was discharged ten days after Lucy's birth, and although I was obviously looking forward to going home, somehow it didn't seem the right thing to do when Lucy couldn't come as well. However, it helped greatly having Emma to go home to; she needed some attention, as she had inevitably been somewhat overshadowed by her sister's unscheduled arrival. When I went into the baby unit before going home, I saw that Lucy's eyes had completely opened, and when I said her name, her eyes moved to look at me. Although she wouldn't have had very good vision, she was certainly reacting to my voice. I felt so close to her then and told her that she had to keep fighting to live. She had to come home.

ten

BACK at home, the reality of what had happened hit me all over again. The pram was there waiting, as was the cot, nappies and baby clothes, but no baby. I became depressed and very anxious, always jumping when the phone rang in case it was the hospital with some dreadful news. We got into the routine of visiting Lucy twice a day; sometimes Ken and Emma would come with me and sometimes I would go alone. I would sit beside the incubator praying and talking to Lucy about anything and everything.

When she was three weeks old, Lucy was allowed out of the incubator for a quick cuddle, which was a wonderful moment in our lives. Although she was still attached to the monitors, she was now breathing independently most of the time. In the incubator her head was inside a bubble like an astronaut's helmet, and this gave her pure oxygen. It was fabulous to hold her, even for just few minutes, and kiss her tiny face.

Emma sat beside me on the first occasion and patted Lucy on the head saying, "She's all right for a sister, Mummy, but she's too small!"

I did my best to assure her that Lucy would grow in time. One morning when Lucy was about a month old and had been

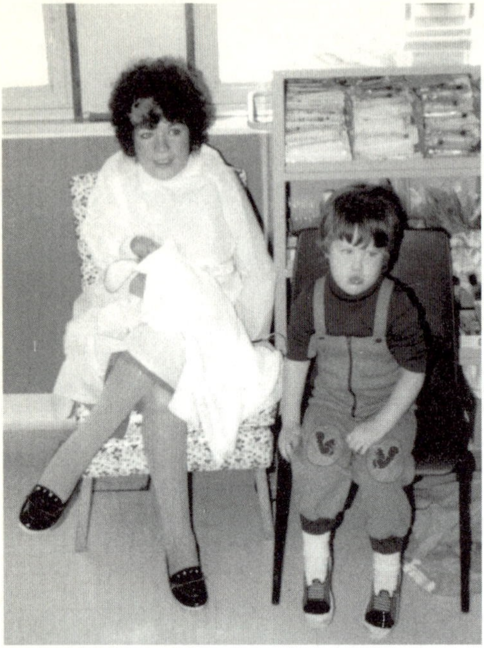

With Emma & Lucy, just before leaving hospital

progressing well, we had a phone call from the hospital, telling us that overnight Lucy had got an infection and was very poorly, and that it would be best for us to go to the hospital at once. Ken was back at work now and Emma was at school, so I went alone. As I drove to the hospital that day I felt sickened by the dreadful apprehension of what I would find when I got there. Lucy had been doing so well, everyone said so in the unit, so why now, when her weight was getting on for two pounds and her milk intake had been increased, had she suddenly got this infection and gone downhill so quickly?

At the hospital I saw that Lucy had been put back onto the ventilator, being too weak to breathe for herself. She was being given a blood transfusion, and the needle was in her head, supported by a plaster cast which looked somewhat like a turban and, I thought, very painful. Her mouth was opening and closing and her face crinkling up as though she were crying, but there was no sound. The lovely pink colour she'd had to her skin yesterday was gone now, replaced by a dull yellow tinge.

I sat down beside her incubator and wondered, for the first time since having her, whether it was really fair to keep her alive like this—what if she were disabled physically or mentally? If she were physically disabled I wouldn't be able to care for her because of my own disability, and what if she had to go away from home as I had? Talk about history repeating itself. If she were severely mentally disabled, in my opinion it would be kinder not to let her live. During my time at Chailey, I had seen a great many children who were so mentally disabled they hardly knew what day it was. I certainly wouldn't inflict that on my child if I could do something about it.

As these desperate thoughts went round in my head, the nurse said that if Lucy could fight off the infection she may well improve. But there were no guarantees, just wait and see was all we could do. I understood then, as I sat there beside Lucy, why the nursing staff in the baby unit would never join me in any optimism when Lucy had been doing so well. It can all change so quickly with these tiny babies, and they had obviously seen many babies not survive. I cried and cried that day; everything seemed so black, and though I tried to reach inside myself for a positive thought, it would not come.

I looked around the unit at the monitors showing the babies' heartbeats, and at the nurses so dedicated to their cause. I watched another mother and father through the glass in the next cubicle, where the babies were promoted once they had put on weight and were out of danger. The mother's face shone with love and, I suspected, relief that the nightmare for her was over, her child having successfully graduated from this most precarious situation.

I closed my eyes as the regular clicking of Lucy's ventilator echoed in my head. I felt so helpless. I had phoned Ken from the hospital and had arranged for our neighbour to collect

Emma from school. That day was one of the longest I have lived through, and when I got home that evening it was difficult trying to explain to Emma about her sister.

I remember Emma sitting on my lap, as she often did, and putting her hands either side of my face, looking into my teary eyes and saying in her straightforward way, "Look Mummy, is Lucy going to heaven or coming home?"

She always took it for granted that I had the answer to any question she asked, but I didn't have the answer to this one. Everything is black and white when you're four years old.

When I phoned the hospital early the next morning I was told that Lucy was "holding her own", that she was no better but no worse. For the next three days while the infection lasted, I sat beside Lucy's incubator and willed her to pull through.

Finally, on the morning of the fourth day, she began to recover. The yellow tinge left her skin and her colour became healthier. The ventilator was removed, as was the needle from her head, and as I spoke to her, she once again reacted to the sound of my voice and looked in my direction. The black cloud lifted from our lives.

Lucy began to gain weight more rapidly as her feeds were increased. Over the next two months, her once skeletal form bloomed into that of a lovely baby. One by one the wires were removed from her body, and after three months she was taken out of the incubator and put into a cot. On the day she was moved into the next cubicle we were ecstatic! The nursing staff were then able to share our joy as Lucy was at last out of the woods.

On the day that she should have been born, 1st October 1982, we took Lucy home. She weighed four pounds. Those three months Lucy spent in hospital were anxious times, but my memories of the nursing staff at the Special Care Baby Unit are very special ones. It is a place of great hope and dedication, and I can never thank the staff enough for the life of my daughter.

Having witnessed Lucy weighing just 29 ounces at her birth, she now seemed quite big to Ken and me. However, apart from a quick visit by her grandparents during her time in hospital, Lucy had not been seen by anyone else. Now that she was out of hospital, people constantly remarked about how small she was when they saw her for the first time. Although we had taken photographs of Lucy whilst she was in the incubator, it was not easy to convey to others just how tiny she had been.

Although it was wonderful to have Lucy at home, the first few months of looking after her were very stressful; despite the fact that she was three months old, she required the care of a new-born baby. She had to be fed every four hours and didn't sleep for very long between feeds.

Ken and I were very tired, and we still had Emma's needs to consider as well. Ken had started a new job which he was quite anxious about, and lack of sleep made him very irritable. I was always careful not to leave him in sole charge of Lucy, as I knew he found coping with fretful babies difficult. If he were to lose his temper with Lucy, the consequences could be dreadful.

We had grown apart during the first years of Emma's life. She was, admittedly, not an easy child, and she would argue with him endlessly. Sometimes he would try to show her how to do something, and if she wasn't able to do it, or to understand what he meant, he became very short of patience. One evening a few days before Christmas, we were all in the lounge and Emma was playing with her Lego bricks. It was approaching her bedtime and Ken asked her to put the bricks away in the tin. Emma, who clearly didn't want to stop playing or go to bed, began reluctantly putting the bricks away, and then tried to put the lid on. She struggled with it for a minute or two and then because she couldn't fasten the lid, her temper got the better of her, and she threw the tin, spilling bricks all over the carpet.

Ken's reaction to this was instant: his hand was at the back of her head and he pushed her face down into the bricks on the carpet, shrieking at her to clear them up again. Emma screamed, and when she looked up at me, I saw she had blood running down her face, coming from a cut in her forehead where one of the bricks had penetrated her skin from the force of the push. I yelled at Ken to get a cloth as Emma rushed to me. There was a lot of blood coming from the wound, and I thought Emma might need stitches in it. I was livid with Ken, but wanted to defuse the situation for Emma's sake, she was frightened enough. So I didn't shout, but tried to keep my voice calm as I told Emma to hold the cloth on the cut, and said that I would take her to the hospital.

As I was getting my shoes on, Ken was saying to Emma, "Daddy loves you, Daddy's sorry." His voice was sickening to hear, pathetic, and he was trying to put his arms around her.

I could hardly bear to look at him, but muttered, "Look after Lucy," as Emma and I left the house. I didn't want to leave my baby, but what else could I do? I couldn't pick her up and carry her to the car.

As I drove to the hospital, my mind in turmoil, it occurred to me that I had now been placed in a very precarious position. Here I was, a very disabled woman, in charge of two small children, with a husband who couldn't control his temper. It didn't take much working out that the Social Services would quickly interfere in a situation like that if they should hear of it.

I said to Emma, who by now had calmed down a little, "We're going to play a game now Em—if the doctor asks you what happened, say you fell."

"But Daddy did it," she sobbed.

"I know, darling,"I said to her, "but we must keep it a secret, so that nobody thinks that I can't look after you properly, and take you away." There was no point in telling her anything but the truth, as I knew that what she told the doctor was so important.

Once we had registered at the hospital, we sat in the children's waiting room. Emma put her little hand in mine, still pressing the now very bloody cloth to her head with her other hand. While we looked at a picture book together, I thought about all the time I had spent in this hospital that year, with Lucy fighting for her life. The days had seemed endless, so many highs and lows, so many prayers and finally, such joy. Now I was just so ashamed, of Ken and the reason Emma and I sat here tonight. When the doctor examined Emma's forehead, he said she would need a stitch or two, but they could use adhesive strips which would pull the wound together. I was so relieved that no needles would be involved. When asked what had happened, I explained that Emma had tripped. Emma looked me straight in the eye, but she didn't contradict me.

Home was the last place I felt like going as we left the hospital that night, it was after 10 o'clock, and Emma was exhausted. When we got home and I was putting Emma to bed, Ken was quiet and I knew he was feeling ashamed of himself. When he said goodnight to Emma, he kept apologising over and over to her, pleading for her to forgive him, saying that it would never happen again. That, at least, was one thing we were both agreed upon. The trouble is that once things have happened, there is no way of erasing them from your memory; you carry them with you for the rest of your life and you just do your best not to consciously think of them too often because they always cause you pain.

Later, Ken and I talked about what had happened, and about all the other times when he had lost control of his temper. I told him he had to go and talk to someone who could offer him professional help, and he would have to be honest about all the times he had been near to harming Emma; about the rage that took him over and why. For the first time he told me that when he was a child, his father was sometimes violent to him and his brothers and sisters. I supposed it was a case of what goes round comes round, and he was behaving to his child as his father had behaved to him. I told him that whatever the reasons were that made him what he was, violence would have no place in the lives of Emma and Lucy. Children do not ask to be born; I believe they deserve to grow up in the very best environment that their parents are able to provide for them.

With the New Year of 1983 things settled down, as they seem to have a habit of doing. As a result of his visit to our doctor, Ken was offered counselling, which gave him the opportunity of unloading some of his emotional baggage. It is not an easy thing for anyone to do, and even more difficult for men who, on the whole, seem to find talking about feelings more difficult than women do. I was pleased that he was willing to seek help.

Lucy was doing well and continuing to gain weight. She had monthly visits to the hospital, where checks were made on her development. It was thought by the doctors there that by the time Lucy was five years old, she would have caught up with her growth and mental development, and there would be no obvious signs that she had been such a premature baby. The doctors, though, were the first to admit that they were still learning about these tiny babies, and obviously each case was very individual.

Having relaxed somewhat since having had Emma, I was happy to accept a little help from Social Services towards Lucy's care. This came about because I wanted to be able to drive

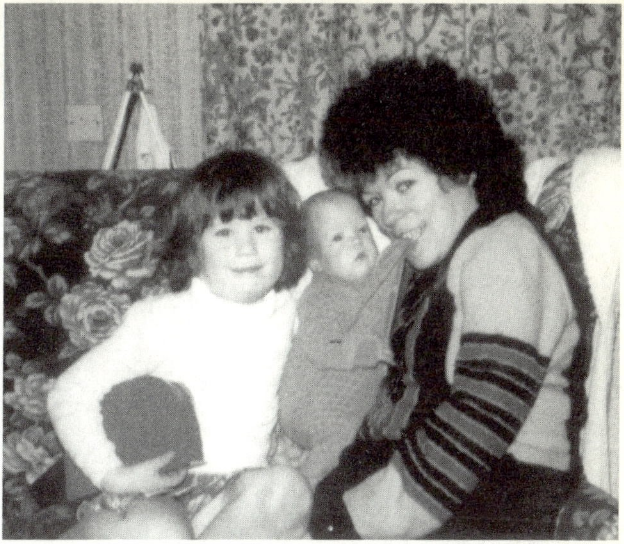

With Emma & Lucy, Christmas in Brighton 1979

Emma to school each day, to keep to the usual routine for her. With Ken at work, there was no way I could get Lucy into the car by myself at that time, so I contacted Social Services, who sent a young lady called Linda to help.

Linda was in her early twenties, and her job title was Family Aid. On her first visit to me she stressed that she was there to do only what I asked her, and nothing else. At first I told her that I only wanted her to sit with Lucy whilst I drove Emma to school, as I wasn't keen on letting anyone share in Lucy's care. However, over the weeks we became friendly, and gradually I grew to trust her enough to let her bath and dress Lucy. She would then leave, and return when it was time for me to collect Emma from school. Despite my friendship with Linda, I was careful what I spoke to her about, remembering always that she worked for Social Services.

Over the next few months Linda grew fond of Lucy, but she never tried to take over or undermine me. During the day when Lucy and I were alone, I loved looking after her. She was still so light that lifting her in my teeth was easy, although I had to be really careful not to lift her up or down too quickly as she was not able to raise her head as soon as Emma had. Dressing Lucy was often more of a trial for me than it had been with Emma, because her arms and legs were so small, but we gradually got used to one another, and as she developed it was wonderful to see her smile and watch her play with her toys, particularly when we had been so close to losing her.

If you have read this book from its outset, you will know that my life has been one of daily challenges, never easy. Often the most fundamental things have been hard to overcome, leaving little room for happiness, and my children have been my greatest joy.

However, since I was ten years old there has been another source of great joy in my life. I first heard a song called *It's Not Unusual* on the radio, and subsequently saw the singer performing it on television. I remember that I was absolutely transfixed as I watched this wonderfully handsome man gyrating around as he sang. I could not take my eyes off him, and from that day on I have adored him.

For me Tom Jones is totally unique, both in the way he looks and sounds, as well as the way I feel about him. I love to hear him sing, and never miss watching when he's on television. At times, when things are particularly difficult, I have only to hear his voice to find comfort in its almost tangible strength. Tom has been part of my life for so long now that I can't imagine it without him. Over the years my feelings for Tom have become a standing joke to those close to me!

You can guess, then, how I felt when I saw in the local paper that Tom Jones was coming to Brighton to do a concert! I just had to go, and Ken agreed to come with me. A friend said that after all these years of listening to Tom's records, I might be disappointed with seeing him live, but I didn't agree, of course.

As the date the concert grew closer, I was really excited; I just could not wait to see Tom in person. Emma didn't understand what all the fuss was about, although she knew it had something to do with the man whose picture was up on the wall (I've always had pictures of Tom up in my home; it wouldn't really seem like home to me otherwise).

The night of the concert finally came and Ken and I arrived at the Brighton Centre. I was sorry that the space allocated to wheelchair users wasn't a bit nearer to the stage, although I had a good view. I couldn't believe that Tom Jones would soon be in the same building as me! There was a comedian on stage first, and then an interval which seemed endless. Then, as the lights went down, an expectant hush filled the hall, and I felt as though butterflies were doing somersaults in my stomach.

Suddenly a voice boomed out, "Ladies and Gentlemen, This is Tom Jones!"

Light flooded the stage, the applause and screams from the audience overwhelming as he came into view. Tom was wearing a blue suit and white shirt, and he looked fabulous. He was everything I had hoped he would be, and his voice was as fantastic live as it is on record. He smiled and waved at the audience as he sang his way through the songs that had made his name in show business.

Each song he sang was so full of emotion, I felt he was singing just to me. It was wonderful to see him standing up there on stage. It reiterated how very dear he has become to me over so many years, and I felt I knew him very well. In between the songs women went up to the stage and he kissed them or wiped his sweaty face on their underwear, as only Tom can do! It was very hard for me not to be able to run up to the stage, and I confess to being quite overcome with jealousy! But there's no room for sadness or regret, not with Tom, and I was so happy to have seen him at last.

I have seen him on many occasions since that first time back in 1983, but more about that later. My favourite of all Tom's songs is called *With These Hands*. It is a love song which Tom recorded way back in the early years of his career, and its words are beautiful. I have dedicated this book to Tom Jones, as well as to Emma and Lucy, for all the joy they have collectively brought into my life. Thank you, Tom.

eleven

LATE in 1983, Ken and I went out for a meal with friends I had kept in touch with from my school days. One in particular, called Phillip, visited our home regularly. Phillip had been born with spina bifida, although he was able to walk with the help of crutches. He didn't work, but photography was a favourite hobby of his, and he took some excellent pictures of Emma and Lucy.

We arrived at the restaurant to see that Phillip had brought along another friend of his, called Graham, who had also been at Chailey with us. Although I remembered Graham from school, I hadn't known him well; he was about five years older than me, so he had left by the time I was starting secondary school. Graham also had spina bifida, and he was more severely disabled than Phillip. Although he could walk, he also used a wheelchair which he found a far more efficient way of getting around.

Graham had been married but was now divorced and had his own flat in Hove. We chatted about the old days at school, and the various characters at Chailey who we had both known. I found him quite attractive, with his very blonde hair and blue eyes, and realised we shared the same sense of humour; we laughed a lot together that evening. He seemed to have organised his life well; he was also a keen photographer, which took up a lot of his time. Graham no longer worked, and as well as photography he was also a keen archer.

After that evening, Phillip often brought Graham with him when he visited us, and I began to look forward to seeing him. We had a great deal in common, for as well as our disabilities, our outlook on life was similar. I could identify with Graham's views and how he coped with his disability; he was very intelligent and I liked being with him. And he was fascinated by Lucy: because of his disability, he wasn't able to have children of his own, so being around them was a new experience for him.

By the spring of the following year, Graham and I knew that our friendship was becoming more serious. His visits brightened my days and gave me something to look forward to. Although I had been with Ken for eight years, I knew that I was no longer in love with him. Subconsciously I didn't want to put my thoughts into words, knowing how much hurt and emotional upheaval it would cause Ken, but Graham and I finally got round to talking seriously to each other about our feelings, and decided that we would like to be together. I said that my daughters and I came as a package: there was no question of me going anywhere without them. Graham accepted that, and said he had never expected anything else.

I knew now that the time had come for me to tell Ken. I had no intention of sneaking around behind his back as though I was having a seedy affair, but I was dreading it. I knew he would be devastated, and there was also the possibility that he might become violent. He wasn't only losing me—to a certain extent he was losing his children as well.

At first, Ken didn't think I was serious when I told him, and he began to laugh, but as he took in what I was saying and realised that I wasn't joking, the laughter stopped. He began asking how Graham and I would manage with the children, how we'd get the shopping, do the household tasks. Then he said that if I stayed he'd change, he'd learn to drive and be more patient with the girls. But although his behaviour had improved since he'd been receiving help from the doctor, nothing would alter my decision.

Finally he became angry, and I was very frightened. I was totally unable to defend myself physically should I have needed to, and I didn't know what was going to happen next. He shouted a lot and threw things, but he didn't hurt me. I knew, though, that now Ken understood how things were, we had to separate as soon as possible. There was no point at all in dragging things out; I couldn't stay and bear the brunt of his hurt.

Ken made it clear that he had no intention of moving out of the house, and I knew it had not once crossed his mind that I would go. But that's exactly what I did, and within a few days, Emma, Lucy and I had moved in with Graham.

My family aid, Linda, was a great help to us with the move and settling into our new life. She was, after all, there to help me with whatever I needed.

Graham's flat was spacious but only had one bedroom, so Emma and Lucy slept in the lounge. Emma thought it was a great adventure, although she was concerned that Ken would be all right on his own, and I did my best to explain the situation to her in a way that she understood. Although I felt some relief that the actual physical split between Ken and myself had taken place, I was forever looking out of the window expecting to see him there; he didn't know exactly where Graham's flat was, but I knew he'd find it.

Ken phoned constantly, begging me to go back to him. I told him that I could never go back, but that I would take the children to him at weekends; there was no reason why he should lose touch with them. I continued to drive Emma to school each day, wanting to keep things as normal as possible in her daily routine. My family thought I had gone mad when I told them about the split. They knew nothing about the problems within our marriage; Ken was always on his best behaviour when we saw them, and I am sure they had been more relaxed thinking I had an able-bodied man 'looking after me'. Naturally, the main thing that concerned them was that Graham was disabled and consequently we wouldn't be able to manage with the children, but sometimes you can't tell people how you'll manage, you just have to show them.

Graham was an only child. His mother lived nearby, and at first she was horrified that her son had acquired a ready-made family. His relationship with his mother had always been a difficult one; he felt that she had never really accepted the fact that she had given birth to such a disabled baby. Over the years she had not neglected him in a material way, but he felt that he had never received the love he craved from her. They got along in a very basic way, but he never felt he lived up to expectations she had of him. However, when she got used to the idea of her son being a family man, she doted on Emma and Lucy.

At 18 months, Lucy could just about sit up without help, and she could stand only by being supported, so I used to hold her in between my knees, which she loved. She wore reins all day as Emma had, so that I could get hold of her. She had no idea about using her potty, and I found it very exhausting trying to teach her about the toilet.

Lucy was still attending the hospital regularly, but it was more to see how she was developing than to provide help; as I have said, the doctors admitted that the development of children born so prematurely was still a grey area for them.

Eventually, Ken moved out of the house in Brighton and Graham moved there with us, giving up his flat which was not going to be suitable for all of us in the long term.

Although the modifications in the house such as the stairlift and the shower were suitable for my needs, Graham found them difficult to use. His disability was very different from mine: he had full use of his arms, but was unable to use his legs at all, which made getting on and off the stairlift very hard for him. Also he had to get his wheelchair close to the stairlift before he could transfer from one to the other, and there wasn't enough space at either end of the stairs for this to be accomplished without quite a struggle. After a few months, we discussed moving to a single storey property, which would make life easier for us all.

I put our name down on the council mutual exchange board to see whether anyone had a ground floor flat or bungalow they would like to swap for a house. Amazingly, within a week or so, we had a phone call from someone who lived in Newhaven, about ten miles from Brighton, which was where they wanted to move to. We went to see the flat, which had a garden, two bedrooms and a very large lounge. The bathroom was on the small side to accommodate a wheelchair, but Graham felt that he would manage. It was by no means perfect, but it was more convenient than what we had. The swap was agreed and in November, 1984 we moved to Newhaven.

I knew that because of Graham's disability I was going to have to be more mobile. Obviously there was no way Graham could push my wheelchair, and I had two young children depending on me. At that time in my life I was able to walk much further than I can these days: although polio is not a progressive disability as such, it is a debilitating one. The main danger of my walking so much was that it increased my risk of falling. Although my falls were by now far more infrequent than they had been in my childhood, they were still awful.

Our flat was in a hilly area of Newhaven, which made life more difficult for Graham as far as getting out in his wheelchair was concerned, and although we did not live far from the town, he had to use his car to get there. My memories of that time in my life are that, both physically and mentally, I worked harder then I have ever done. Lucy was now just over two years old, and taking care of her took most of my time. I no longer had a family aid as Emma's school was situated within walking distance of our house.

Lucy's development was proving slower than I had expected; although she could now walk, she was very unsteady on her feet. She had a cold constantly and was always getting infections on her chest, so we spent a lot of time waiting to see the doctor. On one occasion she was prescribed penicillin, which provoked an allergic reaction. She developed red blotches on her body and got into a furious temper, often clawing at my face. This episode really frightened me; I wondered what was happening to her.

Then when she was about two and a half I noticed that one of Lucy's eyes was beginning to turn inward as though it were going behind her nose. We were referred to the eye hospital in Brighton, and spent many hours sitting in corridors waiting to be seen. Luckily by this time she was able to walk quite well. She still had the habit of toppling over sometimes, so I would hold on to her reins and steer her in the right direction. This was very precarious for me, as when Lucy stumbled I was always worried that she would pull me over as well! I had to watch every step I took and be so careful that I didn't fall; often the waiting room at the hospital was full of children, and there were toys acting as an obstacle course all over the floor. Looking back, it was an absolute nightmare!

Lucy would sometimes have eyedrops to dilate her pupils, which made it easier to examine them. Once the drops had been put in we had to wait 20 minutes or so for them to take effect. Lucy found this quite uncomfortable and would cry the whole time, despite my efforts to comfort and amuse her. Eventually, after many tests, she was found to be severely short sighted. She would need glasses, and in order to help strengthen and straighten her weakest eye, it would have to be exercised each day. This was achieved by putting a patch over her good eye, forcing the weaker one to work harder.

At first Lucy hated this hour each day, but after a while we got into the routine of putting the patch on after she had watched *Playschool* each morning; she would come into the lounge, clutching her Postman Pat toy and say, "Patch time, Mummy." She was a dear little girl, so very precious to me after all she had been through.

Lucy has always loved music, and even at that age while her good eye was covered, she would dance around and click her fingers to the song by Wham called *Wake Me Up Before You Go Go*! I was amazed that, even though generally her co-ordination was not good at all, she could click her fingers in time to the beat of the music.

In order to help with her constant colds, the doctor prescribed a medicine called Ventolin for Lucy to take three times a day. It would also aid her breathing; sometimes she would get short of breath, partly because of the problems with her lungs when she was born. Giving medicine to a child who doesn't want it isn't easy at the best of times, but believe me, when you only have the limited use of one hand, it's really difficult! I obviously couldn't manage to give the medicine on a teaspoon, so I used a medicine cup. This worked well if Lucy was in receptive mood, but if not I used to have to hold her in my legs, making sure her arms were restrained, and tip the medicine into her mouth, usually at the same time that she opened it to protest! I administered the endless antibiotic syrups she was prescribed during the first five years of her life in the same way.

Emma had settled in very well at her new school; she made friends easily and was very happy in her new surroundings. Graham was continuing his hobby of archery, although he was not able to pursue his other interest of photography, because the development of the photographs involved using dangerous chemicals and there simply wasn't enough space in the flat for him to be able to use them away from the children.

When we had been together for a year or so, Graham's health started to decline and he began getting dizzy spells, which made him feel sick. When he had these episodes he would go very pale, and just want to go to bed and sleep it off.

As the months went on it became clear to me that Graham wanted little to do with the everyday care of the children, which made me feel very sad. To be truthful, he had never taken part in their personal care at all, but he had always been pleasant to them and chatted and played with them, and often fed Lucy at mealtimes. Now he was becoming noticeably distant from them; I thought that maybe it was because he felt increasingly unwell, or maybe it was because Emma and Lucy were not his. Graham was, as I have said, an intelligent man trapped in a very disabled body. He had come to terms with his limitations, probably as much as any disabled person can, but he had never before been in a situation where they were brought home to him so savagely.

Graham's disability made it impossible for him to father children. He had been married once before, and from talking to him I understood that the subject of children had been a factor in ending that marriage. Life can be very cruel, and sometimes people are not able to deal with things that it puts upon them. I know from personal experience that, even if you have been disabled all your life, it can be a real struggle getting your mind to accept the things that your body cannot do.

twelve

It was in the spring of 1985 that Lucy began going to playschool. At first she went for two mornings a week, and she loved to bring me home the paintings she had done. When I saw Lucy in the company of children her age, it was obvious that she had some developmental problems: things that were relatively easy for them to learn, such as fitting shaped bricks into their correct shaped holes, made no sense to Lucy.

It is difficult to gauge the extent of learning difficulties in children of such a young age, because all children develop at different speeds. Socially Lucy had no problems interacting with the children, although she didn't have as great a vocabulary as most of the others. This was confirmed when Lucy was referred to a speech therapist, who said that there was every chance Lucy would catch up by the time she began full time school.

I spent as much time as I could reading to Lucy and encouraging her to talk about the pictures in the book, which she greatly enjoyed. At this time I bought her a large cabbage patch doll; it was the size of a toddler, he had bright red hair and rosy cheeks and she called him 'Harry'. Along with Postman Pat, Harry was Lucy's constant companion and she would walk around with them under each arm.

We had been in touch with social services, as we needed help with our shopping and housework. Our new Family Aid was Margaret. She was in her mid forties and a very motherly type, and like Linda before her, she didn't interfere with caring for the children, but would help if I asked. Probably because she was older than Linda and a mother herself, I became friendly with Margaret and confided in her some of the problems I was having. These included Ken and his access to the children (which was always emotionally fraught), Lucy's difficulties, and Graham's reaction to the children.

To be honest, at that time in my life I felt completely overloaded emotionally. I had no friends and no time to go out and make any, so I had needed someone to talk to. What I had told Margaret had been personal information, not things I would have talked about with just anyone.

Because the playschool Lucy attended was funded by Social Services, they took an interest in the children who attended. Each child was discussed regularly at meetings, and representatives from different agencies attended them. Margaret mentioned to me in conversation that a meeting was being held about Lucy, thinking that I knew it was taking place. But I didn't, and there was nothing that made me more angry than the thought that we as a family were being discussed by people who in the main had never met us. When I telephoned Social Services and asked why I hadn't been invited to this discussion about my daughter, I was told that it was not the usual policy to invite parents.

I made it clear that I didn't agree with this policy and didn't want Lucy discussed without being present, and I was told that I could attend the meeting. When I arrived at the Social Services office, at the time I had been given, the meeting had just finished and the various representatives—the doctor, the teacher, and Margaret—were just leaving. Apparently I was to be told what the powers that be thought I should know after the meeting; indeed, had I not been a few minutes early, I wouldn't have known the meeting had already taken place.

I don't know how much of what I had confided to Margaret she had shared with the meeting. But from the look on her face, which was one of extreme embarrassment, I thought it a pretty safe bet that my confidences had been betrayed. I could only assume that, on my arrival at the Social Services department, I was to have been given an edited version of whatever had been decided would be best for Lucy.

I told Margaret that I was very disappointed in her; I had thought her to be my friend, but I was obviously mistaken and was in fact just a job to her. That was the end, both of my dealings with her and of any trust I ever placed in Social Services with regard to my children, and I immediately removed Lucy from the playschool. Margaret came to our flat the following day, apparently to explain herself, but she had known the time of the meeting and the time I had been given to attend, which was half an hour later. Although she knocked on the door repeatedly, I did not let her in, and despite seeing her around Newhaven, never spoke to her again.

My lovely Emma, who was now almost six years old, helped me with the weekly shopping. It was not easy at first; she found it quite difficult to steer the trolley, especially as it got loaded up with shopping, and some of the heavier items were difficult for her to lift off the shelves. But we were a good team, and we managed to do it, although sometimes she would get help from the supermarket staff with packing the shopping. But whatever happened, I would encourage her and talk her through every task, and she would always get a reward of some kind for being helpful.

Because he had lived alone for quite a few years before moving in with us, Graham's immune system wasn't working as it should, which meant that he was now getting all the coughs and colds that Lucy had. This made him very depressed, and over the next year or so, I saw Graham change from the outgoing, interested person I had first known. He would no longer sit at the table and eat meals with us, in case Lucy coughed or sneezed in his direction. He began to resent the time I spent with the children, and I felt he blamed them for his almost constant bad health.

In time, this inevitably caused problems between Graham and myself. We were still able to talk things through, and when we did, I realised that Graham felt as though he were not part of our family, which brought about feelings in him of jealousy, and I believed at the time if we got married it would help him feel as though he belonged.

Looking back on it now, it is obvious that marriage was the last thing our relationship needed; Graham had his own emotional baggage, which weighed him down heavily. I believe that most of his problems had arisen because of the very difficult relationship he had always had with his mother; from what I know of life it seems to me that if we are not nurtured sufficiently when we are very young, we carry the scars around with us for the rest of our lives.

I think that when Graham first considered living with us, the thought of having two children around him was quite appealing. Perhaps he thought it would make him feel more 'normal', as he was unable to be a father himself. However, the reality was completely different from what he had expected. Lucy, after all, had her own problems with her many coughs and colds, and I would have been glad of Graham's help and support. I know that with many stepfathers there is often a feeling of jealousy toward the children because they take up so much of their mother's love. In my experience, however, the love you have for your children is unconditional in a way that no other type of love is; as Graham never felt that his mother had that kind of love for him, he couldn't really relate to it at all.

On the occasions when he felt well, however, Graham would make an effort and play games with Emma. She really enjoyed Ludo and snakes and ladders, although she was always a sore loser!

Graham and I were married in August 1986; it was a small ceremony in a registry office. The real marriage room was upstairs, but obviously Graham and I couldn't manage to get up to it, so one of the downstairs rooms was decorated with flowers and made to look very nice. Emma and Lucy were bridesmaids, and wore pink dresses bought for them by Graham's mother; they looked lovely, and I was so proud of them both. I knew that it wasn't going to be easy, but I so much wanted the marriage to work, and so did Graham.

We had a caravan holiday that year in Cirencester. It was a long drive from Newhaven and we had to take both our cars because with Graham's wheelchair we couldn't fit all our luggage in one vehicle. Once we arrived at our destination we were all very pleased with our caravan, which had been adapted for a wheelchair user, was very spacious inside and had a ramp for wheelchair access. There were amusements for the children on site: Emma and Graham played quite a few rounds of crazy golf together, and there was also a Postman Pat ride that cost twenty pence a go. Lucy spent a great deal of the holiday on that! Trying to get her off it was quite a task—she clung to it, and each time the ride ended she would say "again"! The only way she could be coaxed off it was with the bribery of food!

I did not bother to take my wheelchair, as there was no-one capable of pushing it. Instead I drove around the site and parked as close as possible to the various amenities. For all the difficulties we encountered, I remain very proud of us all for endeavouring to go on holiday when each of us had so much to contend with. But we truly cared for each other, so the effort was worth putting in.

I was almost completely independent now as far as dressing myself was concerned. I always wore trousers with elasticated waists which were easy to pull on, and also managed to dress my top half, having long since discarded my bra because there was simply no way I could independently put it on. I always found them to be the most uncomfortable things anyway! My socks, however, have been the one item of clothing that I have never really been able to put on. With so much to do for Lucy, I had to be as quick as possible when doing things for myself.

A few months after we returned from holiday, Graham decided he would like to get a dog. He had a preference for border collies, having watched them on television herding the sheep. I didn't object to this; although I had never owned a dog, I knew the children would love it, so Graham bought a puppy which he called Kim. She was absolutely beautiful, with blue eyes and grey and white fur, and to begin with Graham took Kim out every day in his car to a nearby park, where he delighted in teaching her tricks.

I was very pleased about this. It seemed to have given Graham something to care for that belonged to him, and they became very close, although I noticed that Graham was always anxious about Kim's behaviour. If one of the children stroked her and she became excited, Graham would say Kim should be left alone. After a while I realised that Graham was not able to share Kim with the rest of the family—he wanted to keep her all to himself.

When Emma asked whether she could walk Kim round the block, Graham always said, "No, leave her." Actually, it is hard to imagine a dog less suited to being cooped up in a flat most of the day than a border collie. They are such energetic dogs, and because they are intelligent, they need constant stimulation—if they don't have it they become bored. A run once a day is not enough for this breed, but it was all that Graham was able to offer.

In 1987 Tom Jones came back to Brighton and I went to see him in concert, with the husband of a friend. This, I hasten to add, was a purely practical arrangement but nevertheless, it was not something Graham was very happy about. He knew there was no point in arguing about it, though: seeing Tom is not negotiable in my life—if he's there, I go. As before, Tom was fabulous on stage and I thoroughly enjoyed myself, joining in with all the old favourites like *Delilah* and of course *It's Not Unusual.* We all need something to give us a break from the problems and monotony of everyday life; nobody should be denied that.

I did appreciate, however, that from a man's point of view, it couldn't have been easy for Graham being so disabled, to have me going on about this big able-bodied man, so afterwards I didn't say more than I needed to about the concert and how lovely Tom Jones was, and how I wished I could be trapped on a desert island with him forever!

Seriously, I had no wish to humiliate Graham or make his life any more difficult for him. At this time I was experiencing great problems with my periods. From the time I had begun them when I was 11 years old, they had been a great difficulty for me each month. It's very difficult, when you only have one hand, to sort yourself out when they are really heavy, and I used to get absolutely exhausted with the effort of struggling. The more I struggled the hotter I got, and then everything stuck to me and it was a complete nightmare. Although they were always heavy, they had become unpredictable after I had given birth to Emma, and consequently I could be out anywhere and I might start an unexpected period. This was really not acceptable, and it was a constant worry to me. Also, it is not something you can ask anyone to help you with, its far too personal. So I went to discuss it with Mr Bostock, the gynaecologist who had looked after me while I was pregnant. He was great as usual, and after discussing it with me, he thought the best thing would be for me to have a hysterectomy, which I had at the end of 1986.

The operation was a great success and I was in hospital for ten days or so. Mr Bostock performed the operation himself and Graham looked after the children with help from a neighbour. Although I missed them so much, I knew that my life would be so much easier, and it was a great relief to know that after the operation, I would no longer have to worry about getting 'caught short' any more.

Lucy started school in 1987. The school was only a short walk from where we were living, and it was at this time that I first used an electric wheelchair. My father bought it for me; it cost something like £1,200 and it opened up a whole new area of independence for me. For the first time in my life, I could go out alone without the worry that I might fall. It was absolutely fantastic, I felt so free and in control. Lucy would walk behind my wheelchair, holding on to the handles when I took her to school. For the first time I was able to chat to other mums who were walking their children to school, instead of just sitting in my car and saying goodbye to my girls from there. It made so much difference to my life—I felt included.

As we went in to the playground, the children would say, "Lucy, you are a kind girl pushing your mummy to school." I often wondered how they thought I got home!

We had another family holiday that year, not travelling so far this time and going to a bungalow in nearby Littlehampton. Although my electric wheelchair was such a blessing for me, it was very difficult for Graham to dismantle and put into my car. The two batteries were very heavy, and there were the back wheels which were in one section with the motors, and they all had to come off before the chair would be light enough for Graham to lift it into my car.

It would take him a good twenty minutes to do it. I used to hate to have to watch him struggle so, especially in view of the fact that his own wheelchair then had to be loaded into his car. This wasn't a problem for him in itself, but he was exhausted after doing my chair first. We decided that if we went on holiday, once we had arrived we would go everywhere in our wheelchairs; that way Graham would not have to repeatedly load and unload mine.

We all enjoyed that holiday in Littlehampton. Lucy sat on the beach making sandcastles for hours, while Emma enjoyed the nearby fun fair, and I remember how happy Graham was. Life was very hard for us, but we had succeeded in doing ordinary things that families do.

We always took Kim with us, as she was no trouble, although there was one incident on that holiday. We were sitting outside a pub having our lunch, with Kim tied to my wheelchair, when another couple, who also had a dog, came and sat at the next table. Now Kim was rather timid as far as other dogs were concerned. She was sniffing around under the table with the other dog, which suddenly went for Kim. I moved back from the table to see what the trouble was, at which point Kim leapt up on to my lap, with her back leg touching the control switch on my wheelchair.

This caused my chair to go round in circles! I frantically tried to instruct Kim to get down, but my instructions were somewhat muffled, owing to me having a mouthful of dog hair! We must have looked an hilarious sight, this wheelchair spinning round and round with a stressed-out border collie on board, seemingly in control of it, and meanwhile I was being suffocated beneath this dog! The children roared with laughter at the episode!

After that holiday in 1987, I can't remember Graham being in good health for more than a few days at a time. He now had the dizziness and disorientation most of the time, and subsequently he seemed to lose all his enthusiasm. His ambition both for his archery and his photography, which had been so necessary to keep him mentally stimulated, were long gone. The doctors didn't seem to know what the trouble was, but they thought it was an inner ear problem, making Graham feel as though the room was spinning around him constantly.

It must have been dreadful for him. Even if you have these problems when you are able-bodied they lay you low, but being so disabled as well, Graham just had to stay in bed. As a result of this, Kim was going without her walk and becoming very hyperactive and anxious, and the atmosphere in our home was very stressful.

As the months passed, and despite not wanting to face it, I knew in my heart that really Graham wanted out. Looking after himself was quite enough for him, and I knew deep down that he would be better alone. I did care for him, but by this time my feelings for Graham had begun to change: it took me all my time to look after my girls, and that was enough for me. I must confess that I was also very weary of being around someone who was so ill all the time, and so depressed and despondent about the future.

thirteen

At the end of 1987 we moved out of the flat into a purpose-built council bungalow in nearby Peacehaven. It was the best accommodation we could have hoped for, with three bedrooms and two bathrooms, one of which was integral to our bedroom and had a walk-in shower. The place was totally geared for wheelchair users; the kitchen was large with low-level cupboards and a special sink that could be raised and lowered according to requirements, and there was also a good sized garden with a patio area.

Unfortunately we only lived here together for a year or so before our marriage really broke down. I then moved out of the bedroom I'd shared with Graham into what had been Lucy's room, and Lucy moved in with Emma. The children and I spent a lot of time in my bedroom; I bought a television, and the girls would love to sit on my bed and watch it with me in the evenings. It wasn't that we couldn't all use the lounge, but the atmosphere wasn't very healthy.

Kim had by now gone to another home with a young couple who had plenty of time and energy to spend on her. This parting had made Graham feel all the more sad: he had really cared for the dog, but she was far too energetic for his capabilities. In the summer of 1987, shortly before Kim went, we had bought another dog, a Staffordshire Bull Terrier, in the hope that it would be company for her and allay her boredom somewhat.

Having seen an advertisement in the paper, we went along to Hassocks, near Lewes, on a lovely summer day in June. We were shown into a barn by a cheerful lady who had bred the dogs. Along with the mother there were six bitches, all red in colour with differing white marks on their coats. We had only been in the barn a minute or so when a particular pup came up to me and sat herself down very definitely at my feet. While the other five puppies came and went from me, this one sat resolutely in the same position, staring up at me with huge brown eyes which seemed to be saying 'Please take ME home'! There was little choosing to be done!

On the drive home the puppy sat on my lap quietly, and although she was very heavy, I did my best to hold on to her. The girls were delighted with her. Over the next few days the puppy made a strange, squeaky sound whenever she wanted something, so we called her Squeaker. She settled into her new home quite quickly; she belonged to all of us and we loved her very much.

Graham had asked the council for a single flat. Divorce proceedings began, and after a wait of ten months or so, Graham moved out to be on his own. Obviously it is not possible to live through such a situation without any animosity at all, but looking back things were kept reasonably civil between us. I was sad that our marriage had failed; this was my second marriage, and I really had wanted it to succeed, but you can only do so much and we had tried our very best to work things out.

I believed that I belonged to my children, who depended on me for everything. Although they were still seeing Ken on some weekends, they were not close to him emotionally and he was not a part of their daily lives. They had no other relatives living near, so I needed to be there for them, as they were for me.

I didn't relish the thought of being a single parent, although in fact that is what I had been since Graham and I had got together. Although I was now 35, I had never been alone in my life: as a child it was impossible to be alone at Chailey, and when I wasn't at school I had been at home where there was always someone around. Now, when the girls were at school, and, more importantly, when they visited their father at the weekends, I would be on my own.

I had made good friends with a lady who lived across the road from me. Her name was Shirley, and she had three young sons who often came over to play with Emma and Lucy. Shirley assured me that she would be willing to help me any time I needed it, which was a great relief as I had been worried about how I would put my socks on!

I became accustomed to being on my own during the day when the girls were at school, although as Squeaker followed

With Squeaker, Peacehaven, 1993

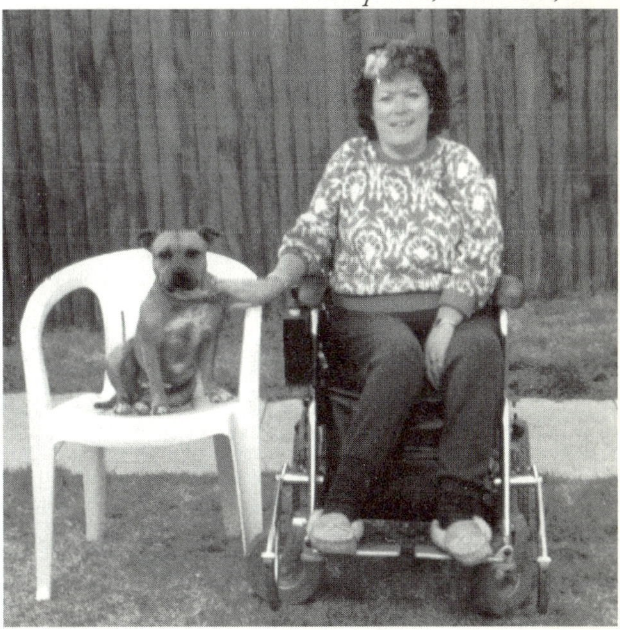

me around everywhere I never really felt alone. She was devoted to me, and I to her. I took her for walks, attaching her lead to the side of my wheelchair, where she would trot along beside me happily. She was a bit too protective of me really, especially if another dog came anywhere near my wheelchair. Then a frown would appear on Squeaker's face and she would growl in warning! On one occasion, she was so desperate to be freed from her lead in order to protect me, that she bit my toe! This only happened once though, which is just as well as Staffordshire Bull Terriers have extremely strong jaws!

So I settled down to life as a single parent. To be honest, it was such a relief, when I woke up each morning, not having to face that terrible, heavy atmosphere which had prevailed during the months that Graham and I were living separate lives in the same home.

I placed an advert in a local shop for someone to come and do some housework for me. Although I could manage the day-to-day tasks, such as the washing and loading the dishwasher, I was not able to do the dusting and hoovering. The advert was answered quickly by a lovely friendly lady called Pat, who was in her late forties, with two boys at school; she lived just over the road from me and had plenty of time for a little job. Once we got to know one another I looked forward to her coming and to having someone to chat with.

I now had to think of a way in which Emma would be able to get my electric wheelchair into my Metro, as obviously I didn't expect her to lift the parts as Graham had done. I began inquiring about various ramps that might be light enough for Emma to lift, and would also take the weight of my wheelchair. If we could achieve this, it would mean that I could take the girls out whenever I wanted, without worrying about Emma having to push me. I would also be able to keep an eye on Lucy, and it would also eliminate any chance of my falling over.

So I contacted some local firms who dealt with such things and, after some trial and error, finally came across two light, telescopic ramps which would fold up and fit underneath my wheelchair in the car. Emma was able to open the ramps, position them at the back of my car and, with practice push my chair up into the car. As there was quite a lip between the back of the car and the floor, I had a false floor made so that when the chair reached the top of the ramp it went evenly into the car.

I don't wish you to think that this was by any means easy for Emma; although she was well built, she was only twelve and electric chairs are very heavy. Each of us, Emma, Lucy and myself, knew that in order for us to be able to do the things that able-bodied families take for granted, such as going on outings, we had to pull together. One thing I know for sure, though, is that adversity brings people very close together, and we drew on each other's resources so that each of us had what we needed. Emma was a star, as she had been when she was a little girl: she was always there for me to rely on.

Lucy was by now eight years old and physically independent, although it was obvious that she still had some difficulties caused by her prematurity. If we were in the supermarket or anywhere that was busy, I noticed that Lucy had a poor sense of direction. She would walk into people, seeming unable to steer herself around them, and even if she had been in a particular place many times, she still wouldn't know the way round. She wore glasses all the time, her eyesight being poorer than at first thought, but in spite of her problems, she was always laughing and singing the latest pop song.

Some of Lucy's problems were to do with poor co-ordination. She had difficulty doing small things with her fingers, like buttoning her clothes, and would often do her coat up putting the buttons in the wrong holes. Although this isn't unusual for a young child, when I pointed out which button fitted which hole, she found it hard to understand the logic of it.

Lucy was having extra help at school, as her progress with reading and writing was proving slower than the other children. Her memory was very short term: if I gave her more then one instruction at a time, she would forget what I had said. She would often put her shoes on the wrong feet, and getting her socks on with the heel in the right place was difficult for her. Over the years Lucy would catch up with these tasks, but at the time I was very concerned about her future.

My neighbour Shirley came over and painted my bedroom for me not long after Graham had left. My treasured pictures of Tom Jones now adorned the walls. After the initial sadness of coming to terms with a failed marriage, I began to feel very good about life and all it had to offer me. I had two lovely daughters and a very suitable home, and I could now get out and about with my children. I joined the Tom Jones Appreciation Society, thus making new friends with whom I had something (or someone!) in common.

Shortly after this, the Appreciation Society arranged a weekend trip to Brussels where Tom was doing a concert. The trip was to take place at the end of April and I had to go! We would be travelling by coach to Dover, and from there by ferry across to Calais, where there was another coach to take us to our hotel in Belgium.

When I sat and considered all this, it did seem rather beyond my capabilities at first: there was no way that I could possibly get into a coach independently, and I knew that I wouldn't be able to take my electric wheelchair. The dismantling of it would be too time-consuming for somebody who wasn't familiar with it.

However, I explained my situation to the person organising the trip, and she said she would find out whether there would be anyone other than the driver of the coach available to assist me. I must confess that I played down the amount of help I would need to get onto the coach, so I'm sure that they probably thought I would just need a hand to lean on. No way—I needed lifting!

My prayers however were answered when I was informed there would be a courier coming on the trip who could help. Emma and Lucy would come with me, of course, and they were very excited about it.

I was really looking forward to the trip to Belgium, but I would lie awake in the small hours of the morning thinking about everything in minute detail. In the days before the trip, I had many such small hours filled with mental pictures of things going wrong, like me being dropped by the courier! Or like Emma not being able to push my wheelchair on difficult terrain and the three of us getting left somewhere.

But for me life is not made up of 'what ifs', it is made up of getting on with things and sometimes taking chances, and these doubts of mine were outweighed by my feelings about how much I wanted to do this. I knew I would never forgive myself if I didn't give it a go, and would always be wondering what it would have been like, had I not gone along with my gut feeling that it would work out all right.

When the day finally arrived, my sister Lynne drove us to Dover, anxiety all over her face.

"Are you sure you'll be okay, Mo?" she asked repeatedly. I couldn't reassure her totally but did my best to calm her worries. Of course I understood her concerns; I was, after all, very disabled, and going to an unfamiliar country with only two little girls to help me.

The coach carrying the rest of the party hadn't arrived at Dover when we got there, and after a wait of half an hour or so, the courier came in to find us. I was rather concerned to see that he wasn't a very well built young man, and I hoped he would be able to lift me. He introduced himself as Martin. He was in his early twenties, quite slim with fair hair and one of the nicest faces that I have ever seen. I was in my manual wheelchair and Emma took me out to the coach which we had to board to drive onto the ferry. My wheelchair was put in the boot and I will always remember standing at the bottom of the steps of the coach, being viewed for the first time by the unfamiliar eyes of the ladies that were fellow fans of the great man as they looked out of the windows. They were obviously surprised by the degree of my disability, their faces told me that, but it was nothing less than I had expected. What makes it so difficult when people first meet a person with a severe disability, is that before you know anything about the person, that is all you see, and the person underneath has to try to make themselves visible.

Obviously this can't happen until they have been given the opportunity to let their personality out, when their disability should become secondary to knowing them as a person. I was greeted by the driver of the coach, a large, friendly man in his mid thirties, who informed me that it was to be his task to lift me on and off the coach.

The door and the steps of the coach were very narrow, making it very difficult for the driver to lift me in the way I had asked him to, which was to put his arms around my middle. After a few unsuccessful attempts to lift me on his own, they decided that the driver would hold my top half and Martin would hold my legs.

That first lift onto the coach was a disaster! My clothes went one way and I went the other! At one point I was being held up by the waistband of my trousers, thinking, "Dear God, please don't let them rip!"

The situation struck me as hilarious, and we all laughed, which helped to break the ice. When finally I got into my seat I was so relieved and I was greeted with smiles and friendly introductions. We soon got chatting—after all, we all had someone in common, didn't we? Martin and the driver assured me they would find a better way of lifting me on and off the coach, and I said that as we got used to each other, things would work out.

After the ferry crossing to Calais, the drive to Brussels and our hotel took about three hours. Throughout the journey Tom's voice filled the coach as his records were played constantly. This helped me when I thought with dread about all the other times I would have to be manhandled on and off the coach. It reminded me that I wasn't going through this for just anyone. No, this was so that I could see Tom.

We arrived in Brussels and settled in to our hotel room, then, feeling hungry, decided to go out and find an evening meal. Emma pushed me, and Lucy was under strict instructions not to let go of my wheelchair handle, I was so worried about us losing her. The roads in Belgium were a complete nightmare to cross. I hated not having the control which I had become used to with my electric wheelchair, but Emma did amazingly well and at last we found a shopping precinct where there was a McDonald's. After burgers and chips, we made our way back to the hotel, exhausted!

We spent the following day at Bruges, a very pretty town not far from Brussels, and by this time we had made friends with a couple of the ladies who were in our party. They were more than happy to help Emma with pushing my chair, and I was surprised at how soon I was accepted. Fortunately, I can get on well with most people, especially if they have a sense of humour. I had a few drinks of Belgian beer that day as well, which was very strong and washed any inhibitions away!

There was a boat trip on offer which I declined—I was having enough trouble getting on and off the coach, never mind getting into boats! However, the girls were eager to go on the river, which they did while Martin took me round Bruges. It was a lovely early summer day, and as we toured the town we looked in the many shops that sold beautiful lace items, as well as many that sold chocolate, which tasted out of this world. Although Martin hadn't had any previous experience with disabled people, he was one of those rare human beings who immediately look at the person you are, not your disability, and I really enjoyed being with him. He was pointing out some intricate work on the front of a building at one point, and when I looked up at it, the sun was in my eyes; whereupon Martin instinctively put his hand above my eyes to shield them from the glare. This kind of consideration is usually only second nature to people who have known me for many years and are aware that I can't lift my arm up, not to someone who has known me less than a day.

When the evening came and it was time to go to the concert, we travelled there in the coach. The driver, who had by now lifted me four or five more times, was getting quite adept: he somehow held me and balanced me on his knee as he walked up the steps (although I had decided that it was safer for me to get down the steps by sitting on my bottom). On arrival at the concert venue, we found that there was a flight of stairs up to the front entrance, and I was aware that most of the ladies on the coach were as worried about this as I was, which I found very touching given that we had known each other such a short time. I heard several voices say, "Oh, look at all those steps," as our coach pulled up outside. From their faces, they were obviously concerned that I would not be able to get in.

"Well," I said, "there's nothing for it ladies, I'll have to go in through the stage door entrance, and who knows who I might bump into!" I did in fact have to use that entrance, but unfortunately, although I had a good chat with the 'roadies' who were busy setting the stage up and putting the equipment together, I didn't come across a certain Welshman!

We settled in our seats, the lights were dimmed, and I was

so excited as first the Blossoms came out on stage. At the time they were Tom's backing singers, three lucky ladies who travelled the world with him, and they began singing *Mr Jones is in town*. I saw the curtain move, and in the dim light made out the silhouette of a man walking on stage. I recognised the figure at once, and though it was obviously a moment or two before he was supposed to be seen, I shrieked his name! Then the lights went up and there he was, smiling and waving as always, as his presence filled the room and his great voice washed over me.

The atmosphere was electric as his body moved to the music, and I was so proud of him—he was coming up to his 50th birthday, and a grandfather twice over! His stamina was amazing; he was magic, and well worth every bit of effort it had taken me to be there with him that night, as for two hours he sang and joked with his audience. I sang along with him to the songs which are, after all these years, like old friends to me: *With These Hands, Delilah, Kiss* and all the rest. My throat was hoarse and I was exhausted after the concert—I always sing louder because I can't clap!—but I was so pleased that I had come on the trip to Brussels; I would have missed so much if I had been too worried about trying new things.

On the way back to Dover the following day, I sat out on the deck of the ferry and watched as Calais became smaller and smaller in the distance. Emma and Lucy were playing nearby, and I was so happy that day; I had such a great sense of achievement.

Later that year when Tom Jones came back to the Brighton Centre, I walked up to the stage. When he was between songs, he knelt down to me, and I explained that I couldn't lift my arm but would love to touch his face. Emma was standing beside me, and she lifted my hand to Tom's face which felt cold and damp with sweat. He took my hand and kissed it and then he kissed my lips! Although I knew what was happening, somehow it seemed surreal, almost as though I was watching it happen from somewhere else. But at last I had achieved it, I had been kissed by Tom Jones and nothing can alter that. What a marvellous evening that was, such a great memory to keep with me, and while obviously I was elated at being that close to Tom, what was so special was that he didn't shrink away from my disability. He could have ignored me but he didn't; he was so natural about it and didn't make me feel any different from anyone else.

fourteen

Now that I was alone during the day at home, I began thinking about doing some sort of voluntary work, as a good way for me to meet new people, as well as getting me out of the house. I wanted to do something that I would enjoy, as well as helping others. I felt I had a good clear speaking voice and would have liked to have been able to work in radio; this would not involve too much use of my hands, my voice being the main requirement. So I contacted the local hospital and asked if they had a hospital radio station. I was told that there was one called Coastway, which was based in nearby Hove and broadcast from a house.

I explained about my disability, making sure the access into the house was suitable for me, and arranged to meet the chairman of the radio station.

The house was terraced with three rooms downstairs, two of which at the back had been converted into studios. There were shelves upon shelves of records and CDs, and I was surprised at all the technical equipment—it really was a bona fide radio station.

The other members, more than thirty in total, were for the most part younger than me, all volunteers and all very dedicated to the cause. They broadcast to hospitals in the Brighton and Hove area, doing request programmes as well as news and current affairs.

The requests were collected by volunteers walking around the wards and asking patients what music they would like to hear. Although I wouldn't have been able to do this without help, I was told that volunteers usually worked in pairs and it was felt that pushing me in my wheelchair wouldn't be a problem. Unfortunately, the hospital radio didn't begin until the evening, which was a shame as it still left my days empty, but my friend Shirley said she was happy to keep an eye on Emma and Lucy during the evening and I would only be doing this once a week to begin with.

I thoroughly enjoyed doing the radio programmes and chatting to the patients. During my time with the station I had various co-presenters, one of whom was Danny. Danny was of Irish descent with classic good looks of dark hair and green eyes and a great sense of humour.

One evening when we were collecting requests, a patient wanted "something from *South Pacific*". Danny said, "How about a bucket of water?" He was great fun and really made me laugh.

Danny would help by putting my headphones on for me before we went on air; he was so relaxed and my disability was never really an issue with him. There was, however, another side to some of the people who were involved in the station: when meetings were held, I felt that the hierarchy would sometimes forget that they were there to provide a service for people, and the egos of the would-be disc jockeys tended in some cases to get rather too inflated.

After a while of co-presenting request programmes, I was eager to do some other type of programme such as current affairs, and invite patients who were well enough to phone in with their views on whatever subject was being discussed. But although I put my case for doing this to the powers that be at the radio station, I was never encouraged to do it.

For the most part though, they were good-hearted people who enjoyed giving their time for free. On one occasion we did a sponsored walk of eight miles from Brighton seafront through to the other side of Hove, to raise funds for Coastway. We all dressed up in different costumes: I was a red Indian and wore a large head-dress with bright coloured feathers. I didn't go in my powered wheelchair, as I was afraid that it might run out of power on the journey, so volunteers took turns to push me along the route, with regular stops to collect money from the various pubs and shops along the way. It was an early summer day and the weather was hot. Emma walked along carrying a bucket into which people threw money, and Lucy, who had insisted on bringing her scooter, whizzed along the promenade until she got fed up with it, at which point I seem to remember both Dracula and Robin Hood having a ride on it!

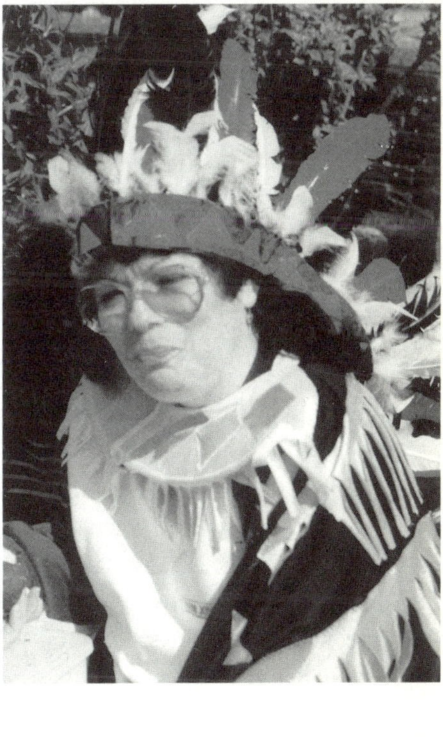

On sponsored walk for Coastway Radio, 1988

There was a huge sense of goodwill and friendship throughout the day. It was great, although on one occasion the person who was pushing my wheelchair at the time let go of it for a second and I found myself hurtling down someone's driveway. I came to rest beside the back garden where its occupants were relaxing, enjoying a quiet summer's day. Their faces took on a very strange look as I came rapidly into view, sporting my red Indian look and roaring with laughter, some of which was slightly hysterical as I was not in control of where I was heading! My small audience gave patronising smiles which said 'poor dear'!

Although I was enjoying being involved with the radio station, I still wanted to do something to occupy my days, so I contacted the Disability Advice Centre for Brighton and Hove to see whether they knew of any other openings for me in voluntary work. I talked to the manager about myself and what I wanted to do, and he said he was looking for volunteers to work at the Centre's telephone Helpline dealing with inquiries from disabled people, their carers and organisations involved with them.

This sounded like something I would be very interested in doing, and after going along to meet Andy, the manager of the Centre, it was agreed that I would work there for a couple of mornings each week. I thoroughly enjoyed my work there; it was a good feeling to be able to give advice and to listen to people who had real problems that I could identify with.

People with many different problems rang the helpline, from people wanting to talk about the feelings of loneliness and isolation that their disability brought about, to those who just wanted advice on where they could obtain a certain piece of equipment. There were always people needing help. A great deal of the information required was available from a large database, which encompassed things like access-friendly holidays, where to obtain wheelchairs, bathing and personal hygiene aids, accessibility of local restaurants and pubs—in fact there was help and advice to be had on just about everything.

When I heard people's stories of desperation it was so satisfying to be able to offer practical assistance. When I felt it appropriate and might help them to understand that I could identify with what they were feeling, I would tell them that I was disabled myself. Andy was a very compassionate person: although he had no disability himself, he was one of the few able-bodied people I've met who can empathise with disabled people and the many problems we have. He really cared about the people who phoned the Centre; it was more than a job to him and he always did as much as was humanly possible to help them.

Sometimes people would come into the Centre to talk face to face, or for help with filling in forms for benefits—these forms are often long and arduous, the questions on them being repetitive and difficult to understand. The correct completion of the form would often dictate whether or not the person received the particular benefit they were applying for, so it was a great source of relief to people that they could receive help and guidance with this task.

At first I wasn't that keen to undertake form-filling, mainly because I felt that, as I write holding the pen in my mouth, it might cause the applicant to lose concentration and deviate from the point of what we were doing, but I felt that I should give it a try. In fact, after the usual "how wonderful" comments, it proved to be quite an ice-breaker. One particular lady was so grateful for my help in completing a form, and consequently receiving the benefit to which she was entitled, that she brought me in a bottle of wine to show her thanks. It made me feel that I was doing a really worthwhile job.

Now that my days were occupied with my voluntary work, I began thinking about my social life. I was 37 years old and didn't relish the thought of spending the rest of my life alone. To this end, I joined a pen pal club and began writing letters to British soldiers, some of whom were posted overseas. I always told my pen friends that I had a disability, usually in the first letter, as I saw no point in not being truthful, especially if I might actually meet them in the future.

Most of the men I was corresponding with were either divorced or going through a divorce, and in some of the letters I received they were quite bitter about their wives, especially if they had children they were separated from. I didn't mind this when I first began writing letters, but after a while it became tiresome to keep reading about so many hard luck stories, as they were all so similar. As well as this, I realised that if they were still carrying so much emotional baggage, they were hardly ready for a new relationship.

Because I had been so candid about my disability when I wrote to soldiers, it seemed to make it easier for most of them to write about it and ask me questions. I felt this was very healthy, and I didn't mind answering them at all. Far better that they should feel able to ask what they wanted to know, than that they should feel embarrassed or awkward, as so many people do around the issue of disability. I am sure that the only way to alleviate this is to talk about it, and for able-bodied people to understand that disabled people are simply people with disabilities. I am not sure whether many of them believed me when I told them that I was writing to them holding the pen in my mouth, although for the life of me I can't see why anyone would say it if it were not true!

Eventually, I did meet two of my pen friends. First there was Rod, who was a sergeant in the Army: we had been writing to each other for a couple of months when he said he would like to come and visit me. I was apprehensive, understandably, because I had not seen a photograph of him and had no idea what he looked like. Whilst I don't really have any particular type of man that I am more attracted to, I hoped he wasn't hideously ugly, or of very small build. I do prefer larger men, probably because they make me feel safe, although the most important qualities for me are that they are kind and that they have a sense of humour—if you can't laugh together, then in my opinion you haven't got much going for you as a couple.

Rod turned out to be about 5ft 11in, well-built, with very little hair. After our initial introductions, which I expected to be stressful, we chatted about our respective children. We had much in common, especially our sense of humour, so we laughed a lot as well! Rod was separated but not divorced, and he made no secret of his hope that he might be reconciled with his wife, whom he thought about a lot and clearly still adored. Because we got on so well as friends, I really didn't mind this and wished him well. I was pleased that he had liked me enough through my letters to bother to come and meet me, and we continued to write to each other regularly as friends.

Then towards the end of 1991 I received a letter from a man called Brian, who lived some twenty miles away from Brighton and was divorced with two teenage sons. Brian had been a paramedic in the Army during his twenty year service and, in common with many ex-servicemen, was now working as a security guard. After writing to one another for a few weeks, we decided to meet for a drink. We had spoken on the phone quite a few times and I liked the sound of his voice (this could have been because he was Welsh, and subconsciously reminded me of another Welshman!).

Our first meeting went well. Brian was well-built, but not so tall that he towered above my five feet. He wasn't particularly good looking; not the type of man I would have looked at twice in the street. However, from our first meeting there was just something about him which drew me to him like a magnet. Maybe it was the confidence he exuded, having lived a full life—he had been in the Army for so many years and had attained a position of authority, Sergeant Major. Another attraction for me was the ease with which he dealt with my disability from the first. He never treated it as a problem when he folded my wheelchair to put in his car, taking everything in his stride. We talked easily together, and were able to be open about our thoughts and feelings.

Brian was very thoughtful of my special needs, always remembering to ask for a straw in my drinks when we were out, cutting up my food after only having been told once that I needed this help, and never giving me cause to feel embarrassed or different. I felt completely comfortable with him. Emma and Lucy liked him too and he had a lot of time for them. He missed his own children, who were living with his ex-wife, although he did see them often. He said he had not known that his wife was going to leave him—she had just gone off to work one morning as usual, never to return.

Just a few days after our first meeting Brian took us all to a fireworks display in Brighton. The girls were very excited. Shortly after we arrived there, Lucy did her usual trick of waiting until we were in the thick of a crowd before she decided she needed the toilet! Despite my worries about having no idea where the toilets might be, Brian took control and carried her through the crowd, assuring her that it was not a problem and making her laugh.

During our time together, Brian took me to the pictures as well as out to pubs and I went to his home regularly. I adored him and couldn't wait to spend time with him: he made me feel so happy that over the weeks I knew him I became totally consumed with him. I wanted to see him, or at least speak to him, every day.

Towards Christmas time that year, when we had known each other for about two months and the highlight of my day had become my contact with Brian, his manner toward me began to cool. No longer did he phone on evenings we weren't together. Although he had always spent weekends in Wales with his family, he had always phoned sometime during the weekend, but that stopped as well.

While I supposed he had begun to feel somewhat smothered by my attentions, my feelings for him were so powerful that they took me over. I had found this man I thought the world of, and I wanted to keep him; he made me laugh, and I really enjoyed being with him, talking to him and having something to look forward to when we were going to see each other. However, relationships are so difficult to get right, and just when you think you're doing well, something goes wrong—at least, that has been my experience.

Eventually Brian told me that he needed some space, a few days when we didn't speak or see each other. Although I told him that I understood how he felt, it was very difficult for me to do. I wanted things between us to grow stronger, not to have to contemplate Brian not being in my life.

It was not to be however, and as happens when feelings are not reciprocal, our relationship came to an end. One evening, after we had arranged that he would come and take me out, Brian didn't turn up. To say I was devastated would be an understatement. I sat by the window and waited for his car to come sweeping round the corner, for him to be standing in the doorway, that ever so confident smile of his spread across his face. His arms outstretched, he would gently pull me to him and I would savour the warmth of him and delight in him being with me. In my mind's eye I reran the scene over and over as I sat in my bedroom staring out into the dark evening. But it would never happen; I would never be with him again. I tried to phone him, but of course he wouldn't answer—if you're going to break someone's heart, you hardly want to discuss it with them, do you?

He wrote me a letter a few days later, saying that he hoped that I would meet someone who could give me the time he couldn't, and apologising for the way he had ended our relationship. Being dumped is never easy; it took me the best part of the next year to get over Brian, during which time I wrote him endless letters (all of which went unanswered), went to his home and just sat outside in my car because I couldn't get up the steps at the front of his house without help—I suppose I just hoped that he would see me and come out and talk to me.

These actions, I know, are totally without logic, but love makes us do bizarre things. Looking back at it now I regret that I behaved in such a pathetic manner, but I was utterly desolate for a while. However, going through so much pain made me grow emotionally: now I guard my heart well. I learnt from that experience, and I will never let another person get to me in that way. I'm worth more than that.

My father had been unwell for some years, and we had learned that he was suffering from cancer. He only found this out when he complained of feeling unwell, and a visit to his doctor confirmed that he had a broken collar bone. He had no idea how this had come about and was most surprised. Subsequent visits to the hospital confirmed that he had myeloma, or bone cancer.

He began treatment and had regular chemotherapy, which caused him to lose his lovely thick black hair for a while. As I didn't see him every day, I noticed his deterioration more than the rest of the family, and when I visited my parents it was sometimes very hard not to break down in front of them. However, knowing how upsetting this would have been, especially for my father, I never did.

It was dreadful to see what this disease did to him, and although everyone shared the secret dread of what the outcome would be, the inevitability of it can never really be dealt with until it happens. You never give up hope in the beginning; I remember my father saying to me shortly after he had been diagnosed, "I'm going to beat this, Mo," his great optimism shining out from his dear face. He was in his mid-fifties then and had recently sold his car breaking business, which had left him financially secure. He was looking forward to spending his retirement years with my mother and enjoying his family: he now had seven grandchildren, all of whom he adored.

He had been able to buy a house near to the town, where my mother had always wanted to live. After years of lugging shopping bags on and off buses, life should have been very good then for my parents: it's what they deserved. But as we all know only too well, we seldom get what we deserve.

In truth, what lay ahead of them were so many hospital appointments, so many days sitting in hospital waiting rooms to have my father's blood tested, and facing the consultant apprehensively for the results—sometimes good, sometimes not—that he was gradually worn down by it.

After a year or so of having treatment, I wondered whether he only continued having chemotherapy as long as he did for the sake of his family, to give us some hope which he didn't have himself. My father was a devout Catholic; he couldn't understand why God had let this happen to him—he had been a good man, had looked after his family, had been a church-goer. When the priest visited him at home, my father's question to him, "Why has this happened to me?" went without answer. There wasn't one.

Having retired from his job in the railway works at Ashford, my father had worked full time in his car breaking business, and had built up a strong reputation as a hard-working man. He knew so many people, being such an outgoing sociable man always ready for a chat, and his hearty Irish laugh would ring out when he shared a joke. He loved to laugh: it was a wonderful sound and I'll always miss it.

In the six months or so before he died, my father deteriorated so much that he had more difficulty in walking than I do, a dreadful thing to witness. My heart went out to my mother who, being a woman of the thirties, had no independence away from her husband and had looked to him for everything. There are no words that can help at such awful times, but we are a large family and we sought comfort from one another.

My father was admitted to the Pilgrims' Hospice in Canterbury in June 1992. I regularly drove up to from Brighton to visit him, sometimes twice a week. I would sit beside his bed and read his newspaper to him, his eyesight having failed because by now he had a tumour in his head. I would hold his hand and chat to him, and sometimes when he wasn't very lucid in his mind he would say that he was coming home and tell us to get him a taxi.

A few days before his death, Lynne, my mother and I sat with him while the hospice priest said Mass and gave Communion. It was one of the saddest, most poignant days of my life, only matched in its sadness by my father's death three days later. Lynne had phoned me to say that my father's condition had worsened, so I drove to the hospice and sat beside his bed all afternoon, watching him while he slept.

His hair had grown back since he no longer had chemotherapy, and was almost untouched by grey. Now and then he opened his eyes; they had that haunted, blank look seen in people worn down by years of suffering, and although in his mind he was confused, I hope he recognised me as I spoke to him and reassured him as best I could. My thoughts drifted back to my childhood, to those precious evenings when he would carry me out to the garden and show me 'Mr Moon' surrounded by his beautiful stars. Sometimes my father would tell me that he had found me in a box in the snow when I was a baby. I loved to hear him relate how he had brought me home to take care of me. How perfect everything had seemed then in my life; the painful truth that parents won't always be around never crosses such a young mind.

Later that afternoon, the nurse began administering morphine injections to him, and he would not know any more. I sat with him, with Lynne and my mother, until he passed away in the early hours of the morning of the 18th June. He was sixty years old. Although at first shock prevented me from registering that I would never see him again, to a certain extent numbing the grief that was to follow, I was relieved that my father's suffering had ended. It had taken five years from the time he was first diagnosed with cancer until his death. If there is a God, I hope my father can see him, because no-one deserves to more.

Prayer For My Father

May the angels take you to their hearts
And lead you
Through a garden full of beauty and tranquillity
May the Lord
Take your hand
Give you comfort and
End your suffering
And may you always know
How very much
I loved you

June 1992

fifteen

IT had been a very difficult year in 1992. With the death of my father my family had been devastated, and my mother was totally bereft. Knowing there was nothing to say that would do anything to ease the huge sense of loss or to comfort her left a feeling of helplessness. Although he had now died, it seemed impossible that he would never again be there beside her; she would talk about the years of his illness, going over and over the treatment he had been given, repeatedly asking herself unanswerable questions: was it the best he could have had? Was everything done for him that could have been done?

Her grief was overwhelming. As one of his children I know how dreadful we all felt when we lost our father, we all loved him so much. But to lose your husband after forty years of marriage must be like losing half of yourself. Her children were my mother's only source of comfort: just talking about our father, sharing our memories of him with each other, sometimes laughing at the things he used to do when he was well.

We remembered the time when he was driving the family down to see me at Chailey when I hadn't been there very long. My parents didn't have much money to buy petrol, so in order to conserve the little they did have, my father would switch the engine off while they were travelling downhill,

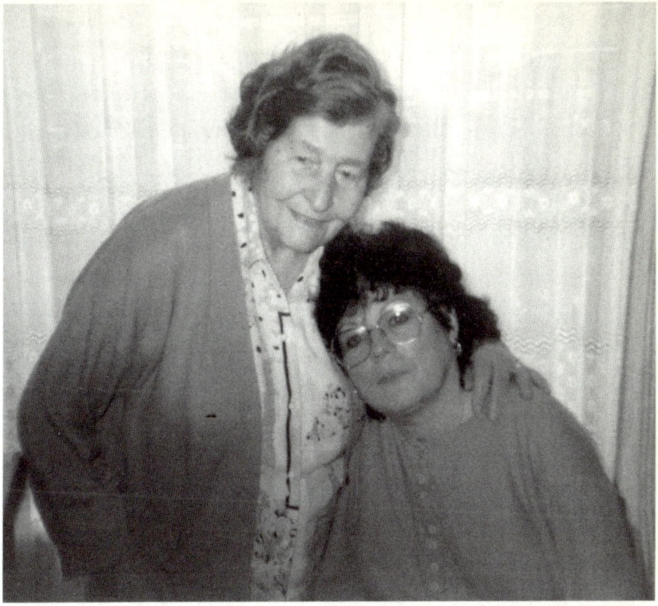

With my father's mother in Ireland

quickly turning it on again before the road turned uphill! On another occasion when his car wouldn't start, he stood alongside it, pushing it in order to get it going while someone steered it. As the car gathered speed, my father realised that he had got the sleeve of his coat caught up in the door handle and ended up running along faster and faster before he could detach himself! As children we all roared with laughter at this spectacle, as did my mother. Recalling these moments, and the years before he became ill, was very therapeutic for us all.

The events that happened after meeting Brian had largely taken away my interest in meeting men with a view to a possible relationship, and I had for the most part given up writing to pen pals. I still wrote to Rod on a friendly basis, as we had established an easy friendship. However, my name must have still been 'on the books', because in October I received a letter from a man called Jeff, expressing an interest in writing to me.

At the time Jeff was still married, though living apart from his wife. Like myself Jeff had been married twice and had two children, although he wasn't in touch with either of them. He was my age, and sounded lonely. I wrote back to him, though my letters made it clear that I wasn't looking for anything other than friendship. I told him about Brian and wrote candidly about how that whole episode had left me feeling.

Jeff lived in Luton and worked as a security guard, but had previously worked in the Territorial Army as a gun fitter. From his letters it seemed that he was a simple man, not in terms of intelligence, but he had simple aims in life, wanting only to settle down with someone and enjoy family life. In spite of my reticence, his letters made that clear.

We wrote regularly over the next few months, learning a lot about each other. I found it a great medium for getting my personality and views across, without my disability being uppermost, which is naturally enough what happens when I meet someone face to face for the first time. I had explained to Jeff about my disability in detail, although he was still surprised when I told him that I wrote holding the pen in my mouth! I always wanted to be truthful about my situation, but at the same time it is very difficult to describe my disability without frightening people away, especially if that person has, as in Jeff's case, no prior experience of it.

I went home to Ashford that year for Christmas. The whole family spent the day together, the first Christmas Day without our father. We drew strength from one another and somehow got through the day, each of us only too aware of the emptiness in the house that only Daddy could fill, never foreseeing a time when we might become accustomed to it.

I was visiting my mother once a fortnight, but it was difficult to stay overnight because of the stairs. When I was younger it hadn't been too difficult to sit down and go up the stairs on my bottom, but now in my late thirties my legs were not as strong as they had been, and the effort had become too great. It was my wish now to move from Brighton to Ashford so that I could be close to my family, though I was under no illusion that it would be easy to achieve. I had no money to buy a property, so I only had two options.

The first was a council exchange, which meant literally swapping homes with someone who wanted to move from Ashford down to Brighton. The council rules for this option required that the person with whom I swapped homes would have to be disabled, qualifying them to live in a property adapted for a person with a disability. This requirement made the likelihood of finding such a person almost impossible, but I put my name down on the relevant form and waited.

The second option would be for me to be recommended by my council in Brighton to Ashford Council for what was called the mobility scheme. This was operated by councils mainly to help people who wished to move to another area for work, as well as for family reasons. But as they only recommended about ten people each year, I didn't hold out much hope that my name would be put forward.

Ashford was fast changing from the small market town it had been in my childhood to a thriving, busy place. The Channel Tunnel was under construction and many people wished to move into the area for employment. I did wonder whether my mother might consider moving from the three-bedroomed home she had shared with my father to a bungalow, where it would be easier for me to visit and spend weekends with her. However, this was never really discussed, as it became clear that she wished to stay in the home that held so many memories of times she had spent with my father.

At the end of January 1993 Jeff came to Brighton to visit me. Although I had seen a photo of him, I had joked with him over the telephone that if I didn't like the look of him when I opened the front door, I would say "yuk" and close the door! I did this anyway when he knocked on my door for the first time, just for the hell of it, but I wasn't disappointed. He was about 5' 9" tall, with greying hair and a thick moustache that gave him a distinguished look. He was of stocky build with broad shoulders, and he smiled when I said hello.

We went into the kitchen and opened the wine he had brought with him. Emma and Lucy came in and introduced themselves amid involuntary embarrassed giggles, whilst Squeaker, my bull terrier, performed her usual party piece of rolling onto her back hoping for a stroke and making sure she wasn't overlooked. After the initial hour or so, we began to relax in each other's company, and Jeff watched while I made a cup of tea. I was a bit embarrassed, as I always am when people watch me do things for the first time, but Jeff soon put me at ease.

He told me that his first wife had left him for another man, and in his second marriage he had been stepfather to four children, who were still in contact with their natural father. Over the thirteen years or so of this marriage, divided loyalties, on the part of both the children and their mother, had been the cause of many problems. Jeff seemed to carry a great deal of emotional baggage, but it was clear from what he said that, despite his past experiences, he was eager to meet someone with whom he might form a successful relationship.

We talked a great deal, and his first visit, which had been planned just for the Sunday afternoon, turned out to last for four days! We were content together, and the children seemed to really like him, which is why he ended up spending his days off work with us. After taking the girls to school we spent one day in Eastbourne just sitting by the sea and chatting. I was really happy and felt so relaxed with Jeff. He had a little experience of handling wheelchairs, gained during the time his mother was dying of cancer. During our first four days together we also visited Brighton, a place I always enjoy going to because of its great atmosphere and history, and its many shops and attractions, including of course the Palace Pier.

And let's face it, there's nothing like eating chips out of the paper and getting your fingers greasy! Although this is difficult for me to manage, Jeff was quite comfortable with feeding me mine. One of the reasons I was attracted to him initially was the ease with which he helped me because it made me feel so ordinary, so normal.

Our evenings were spent watching TV and chatting together with Emma and Lucy; there was so much to say, so much to find out about each other. Emma seemed to like Jeff. At the time she was attending karate lessons in the nearby community hall, and she was eager for Jeff to go with her and watch her practice. I really hoped that Emma would be able to build a friendship with Jeff, because she had never had a successful relationship with a man, and consequently her opinion of men was not very high. Graham had never been close to her, and her father had left many internal scars on her.

Neither of the girls saw their father any more by this time. He had been visiting them every three weeks or so and taking them to his flat in Brighton, which was difficult for us all, because they didn't really want to go. However, they were now old enough to make their own decisions, and they had decided that they no longer wanted to see him. Jeff, however, seemed a person whom Emma was happy to be around, and I had great hopes for the future.

Once Jeff had gone back to his home in Luton I really missed him, as did the girls. Although I was aware that what I felt for him wasn't the same as I had felt for Brian, I was glad about that. I didn't spend every spare minute thinking about Jeff, longing for the phone to ring and to hear his voice; there was no great anxiety in me about how our relationship might develop, it was altogether calmer and, most importantly to me, I felt in control.

Both Emma and Lucy were keen to see Jeff again. In fact Emma was already talking about him coming to live with us, and although it had only been a brief period we had shared together, we had written for some months prior to meeting and things had gone so well that I didn't see the prospect of Jeff living with us as impossible.

As anyone who has had a relationship knows, the first few weeks are very heady times when everything is new, and if you have spent much time alone and have been lonely, it is lovely to have someone to share your time and experiences with. Jeff was eager to visit us again; he phoned me regularly during the first week after his visit and at the end of this time he returned. We were all so pleased to be together again, it just seemed right that he should come and live with us, in spite of the short time we had known each other. Sometimes in life you have to take a chance: if you see a situation that you think will bring you happiness I think you should grab it—there is so little happiness about, and certainly in my life there had been comparatively little.

We discussed the subject of Jeff finding employment initially, but it became clear that financially we would be better off if Jeff didn't work and instead became my carer. We would get an additional benefit, and I would retain the support I already received which entitled us to housing benefit.

I have always felt it to be wrong that when a person receives income support they are prohibited from working more than 15 hours per week and earning anything more than £15, so that they are discouraged from doing part-time work. Such work would earn them additional money, as well as giving them the satisfaction of knowing that, even if they have a disability which prevents them from doing a full-time job, they can still work part-time to give them a feeling of self-worth, of taking part. I would certainly have loved to be permitted to look for a part-time job once Lucy and Emma were both at school, instead of being told that if I wanted to work and retain my benefit it would have to be on a voluntary basis only.

Don't misunderstand me, I know that volunteers are very worthy people, and there is a great need for their services, but for people whose circumstances dictate that they cannot work full-time, the option of working for however many hours they are able should in my opinion be financially rewarded.

I continued my work at the disability advice centre twice weekly; it was important to me and I felt I was doing something really worthwhile in helping people with disabilities. I no longer worked at Coastway Hospital Radio, however, as they had moved premises and the new location was not wheelchair accessible. Meanwhile, Jeff, who was a keen fisherman, would sometimes spend most of the day out pursuing his hobby.

The first few months of us all living together passed uneventfully. We settled down together into a routine, life was good and we were very happy. Then I began to notice what was at first a subtle change in Emma. She was now 14, an age when children embark on that most difficult of journeys, the wilderness between childhood and adolescence, when we seem to be at odds with the world and the people we love most appear to us to be alien to our every thought and deed. There is a distance between us that we cannot bridge, although somewhere lost within our souls, we would dearly love to. We would never admit it though, not even to ourselves because that wouldn't be 'cool', and whatever else we may or may not be in our adolescent years, we must be seen to be cool.

Emma became moody and withdrawn; the eagerness with which she had regarded my relationship with Jeff was waning and any hopes I had harboured of her having a positive relationship with him were fast disappearing. Jeff had for the most part taken over the cooking, which I was quite happy about. It was much easier for him to do it, and I knew that if I had to do it I could. I no longer felt that I had anything to prove to anyone, least of all to myself.

For the past four years I had looked after my children and myself with no other help than having my housework done. Obviously during that time, prior to Jeff coming, the closeness which Emma, Lucy and I had shared had been absolute; and now that the novelty had worn off, it seemed that Emma thought him as somewhat of an intruder into our lives. We had only had each other to consider, and Emma, albeit sometimes without much enthusiasm, had been my mainstay, the person I had relied upon in most circumstances to help me. Every Tuesday after school, we had done our week's shopping, and although she had often moaned about having to do it because she wanted to listen to music or do something else, she had always been there for me. Together we would have to look after Lucy, making sure she didn't wander off or become separated from us. We were a very solid unit, bound together by our deep love for one another and reinforced over the years by so much adversity. Basically Emma was my arms: she was so finely attuned to my needs that most of the time she would just do things without me having to ask her. She was my star in what had been, for the most part, a dark sky before she was born, and her happiness was as important to me as was my own. So it was difficult, to say the least, when the changes in her began.

I suspected that she was feeling jealous of the help that Jeff now gave me; that despite her protests when she had wanted to do something other than help me, there had been a certain comfort in knowing that she was so needed. I think she felt threatened by the fact that there was now another person to help, rather than feeling pleased that she was not alone; and as time passed there was a resentment bubbling away inside her for which she felt guilty but unable to control.

I saw this as quite understandable and tried to discuss it with her, but because feelings on all our parts were so powerful, it was not easy. Sometimes when Jeff put a meal down in front of Emma she would not eat it, saying that she didn't like it, though I knew perfectly well that she'd eaten the same food many times before. Then she became a vegetarian, which meant we had to buy different things for her to eat, and sometimes she wouldn't even eat that. Whilst Jeff was patient up to a point, he is not good at putting over his feelings in a situation that is tense, and when this had been going on for a while he became angry. Then we would have a situation where both Emma and Jeff were angry and I was in the middle, hoping not to be seen to be taking sides.

Another bone of contention between Emma and Jeff was the fact that he smoked: Emma began to object to him smoking in the lounge, so when he wanted a cigarette he would go into the bedroom. Given a choice in the matter, I too would have preferred it if he didn't smoke, but he had done so all his life and it hadn't been an issue prior to this change in Emma. I knew in my heart that although Emma had been so enthusiastic originally for Jeff to live with us, she had now changed her mind and would really prefer it if he left. When, during a talk I had with her, she virtually admitted this, I explained to her that you can't just pick people up when you want to and throw them away when you don't, but it was becoming so difficult to reach her in conversation. She became arrogant, and I was sad to think that this arrogance was hiding so much unhappiness.

Hindsight is a wonderful thing, and I realised that perhaps we allowed things to move along too quickly between the time when we first met Jeff and the time he moved into our home, although because I had been writing to him for some months prior to our meeting, I felt that I knew him quite well. Indeed, once his letters had been arriving for a few weeks, Emma herself requested that she should write to him and I remember one occasion, when he sent her a letter in reply, she positively gloated over it!

I also knew that, in the natural way of things, there would be a time when my children were grown up and would leave home to pursue their own lives, and it is difficult to know just how much we should let our children influence what we should do with our lives. I was still a comparatively young woman at 38, and although my daughters were, and still are, more important than anything else to me, I had a life to live and didn't particularly want to go through it alone. I am not of the opinion that just because I am severely disabled, my children should feel that they have to stay with me rather than do the things they want to. This was one reason that I had been feeling more relaxed about the future, with any constraints Emma may have felt upon her being removed because Jeff was around.

Time passed and Emma began going into Brighton with friends. Of course I always worried about her, especially at night, and didn't relax until I heard her coming in. She began receiving lots of phone calls, always from girls, none of whom I had met or knew of; and when I asked her about her nights out, she was very secretive.

I worried that she was drinking, and about all the things mothers worry about over their teenage children. Despite my hopes that Jeff's arrival would enhance our family, it appeared to be driving us apart. He felt awful about how things were turning out, and although he wasn't nasty to Emma, he didn't have much to say to her—I suppose he didn't know what to say. He had been in a similar situation in his last marriage, which had left him feeling quite insecure, so sometimes instead of trying to talk things over with Emma he would become very quiet.

Maybe this was because he felt out of his depth. All I knew

for certain was that he and I had to try and deal with the situation as a couple, talking about it and trying to understand each other's point of view, or our relationship would not survive.

Meanwhile, dear Lucy seemed for the most part oblivious to what was happening; she was ten years old and her priority was watching *Neighbours* on the television and listening to music. At the time she was devoted to Kylie Minogue, who was in *Neighbours* as well as being a pop star. Lucy loved listening to Kylie's songs and she would sing along and dance around her bedroom. She was a lovely little girl who had overcome so much; and in spite of her problems with learning, she was coping in a mainstream school with extra help. She had lovely curly hair and was always smiling and very loving.

When the time came for Lucy to leave primary school, I was concerned that she shouldn't attend the large school where most of the other children in her class would go, because I knew she would not be able to cope or compete in a class of over thirty children. Also, she would be required to carry books from lesson to lesson, and run upstairs amid the crowds of other children whose co-ordination was far better than hers. I knew she would fail in that situation, so I requested that she be considered for a school that catered for children with learning difficulties, which meant that Lucy had to be statemented. This involved her seeing professionals such as psychologists and doctors who would assess her abilities. The results of their assessments and tests would determine whether she would get a place in a more suitable school for her needs.

Not surprisingly the tests confirmed that Lucy's abilities were below those of her contemporaries, and when she was eleven she went to a school in Lewes, some ten miles away from home. The school was called St Anne's, and Lucy was taken there by taxi each day, paid for by the local authority. As well as children with learning disabilities, there were also children at the school who had behavioural problems, which meant that Lucy sometimes witnessed events she found frightening, like chairs being thrown and shouting and swearing at the teachers.

When we discussed it at home, I explained to her that not all children were lucky enough to have a good home and loving parents, and that sometimes it made them very sad and angry. She understood this and agreed that she would rather be somewhere her problems were understood than in a huge school where she felt completely lost. These outbursts didn't happen every day, and the staff at St Anne's were trained to deal with them. The classes consisted of not more than ten children and there were at least two adults supervising, which meant that the children got more attention and thus were able to progress at their own pace.

Lucy became a very popular pupil and I'm happy to say she thoroughly enjoyed going to school there. As with all the schools my daughters attended, I was made very welcome, and access was always found for me when I went to see the school plays or attended an open day. There was always a space reserved for my wheelchair, and I found the teachers very helpful indeed.

sixteen

NOT long after Emma had turned 15, things came to a head. Her behaviour had continued to be of great concern to me; I knew that something was making her very unhappy, and by now I suspected it was more than the situation at home. I asked her outright what the problem was, and I can still remember the look on her face as she answered me. There was a certain defiance there, maybe even a touch of arrogance as she stood in the doorway of the lounge and said, "I'm gay."

For a moment I couldn't speak, I was so stunned. I think I said something like, "Oh, don't be silly, it's probably just a stage you're going through."

Emma began to cry, and I wondered whether I had misread the look on her face—maybe it hadn't been defiance, maybe it had been fear. It can't have been an easy thing to admit to her mother. It certainly wasn't an easy thing to hear and I didn't want to consider the events that may have taken place, that had brought Emma to this conclusion about herself. She had been spending a lot of time in Brighton, and now that she had broken this news, the phone calls which she had received—all from girls—began to make sense in my mind.

I felt wrecked, and didn't want to discuss it, so devastated was I by what Emma had said. All that kept going through my mind was the same question—why? Why was this happening, why was my beloved daughter being so cruel to me? She must have known how dreadful it would be for me to know that she was gay. I knew that people took a different view on homosexuality in these 'enlightened' days, and to be honest I couldn't care less about most people's sexual preferences, but I didn't want my daughter, my precious Emma, to be a lesbian. I couldn't think of anything more awful happening to our family.

In those first few weeks after Emma had broken the news to me, the atmosphere in our home was more strained than ever, and as though to compound her news, Emma went out and had her shoulder-length hair cut off. Her head was all but shaved at the back, and she began to wear men's suits, which she got from jumble sales and were usually too big for her. She decorated the walls of her bedroom with pictures of women in various stages of undress, and when she wasn't in her room, she spent more and more time out of the house. She was now in sixth form college, almost at the end of her schooling, and she was always worried in case any of the other children at college knew that she was gay. Children can be so cruel, and had they known that Emma was—or thought she was—gay, she would have had a truly terrible time.

Emma had no definite ideas about what she wanted to do with regard to employment, but she had a part-time job in Sainsbury's where she worked on Saturdays and some evenings. The gulf between Emma and myself grew steadily. When I looked at her I couldn't believe that it was the same girl I had brought up. Where had Emma gone? What had happened to her that could have brought about this change? I knew that teenagers could be difficult, but Emma had changed so radically in so short a time.

It would be untrue to say that this situation with Emma didn't cause major problems between Jeff and myself. He seemed to be totally against Emma now, because of what she had done to her appearance and because he had no idea how to deal with her. He was angry with Emma because of the arrogant manner in which she was parading around, and because he loved me and could see how hurt I was.

Sometimes I wondered whether Emma had invented all this to punish me for not telling Jeff to go when she had decided she didn't like the idea of him living with us, then sometimes I would think she may just be craving my attention—most of which she had always had, sharing it only with Lucy. I felt very alone with all this trauma.

I discussed it with Lynne, who was also of the opinion that Emma may just be wanting to shock me, to get attention. Sometimes I would try and discuss things with Emma, about how she felt, and tell her that I still loved her very much whatever happened; but then Jeff would say I was encouraging her to be gay. I tried to explain to him that whether I encouraged her or not, if Emma was gay then that was the way she would be. I knew that he was feeling very insecure amidst all this upheaval, and sometimes I was so emotionally exhausted from it all that I didn't have the strength to allay his fears.

Jeff had asked me to marry him, but I had not been keen—not because I didn't feel enough for him, but because I couldn't really see the point. In my opinion, if you are not intending to have children then there is little difference in being married or living together, but Jeff felt that our relationship would be somehow more cemented if we were married. As we had both had two previous marriages which had ended in divorce, I was surprised that he wanted to get married again. I said to him that we should just see how things developed and not hurry into anything, and what with all the other stuff that was going on I couldn't really think about anything other than Emma and how things were going with her.

However, the months passed and things settled down somewhat. I began, as much as I could, to try to accept that Emma may well really be gay. She had never had a successful relationship with a man; her natural father had hardly been a favourable role model, and Graham had no real idea of what being a father means, and how important it is to a child's future that you make as much as a success of it as is possible. In those circumstances, I couldn't blame Emma for not having any time for men—she had been given no reason to. I know that in many cases, children who admit to their parents that they are gay have been thrown out of their homes and abandoned by their families; maybe deep down the parents believe they have failed their child in some way, and the reason that their son or daughter is homosexual is that they themselves have gone wrong in their bringing up of the child.

All these thoughts crossed my mind at some point. Emma had always been a tomboy as a child; she had hated wearing dresses and had loved nothing more than climbing trees, and had always been more comfortable wearing shorts or trousers. I had never thought anything of it, as lots of girls who are tomboys grow into feminine women. Basically, Emma's homosexuality just left me feeling overwhelmingly sad. It is not for us as parents to decide how our beloved children will conduct their lives, to make choices for them. When they are adults we have to stand back and hope that what we have taught them during the years they were growing up will enable them to be decent human beings, but it is the hardest thing in the world to let go. I knew that, whatever else Emma would or wouldn't be, she had a good, loving heart and that during her formative years she had been surrounded by love.

Jeff and I were married in October 1994, almost two years after he had come to live with us. Our relationship had been more than a little stormy at times, but with the tough issues we had been faced with, that was hardly surprising. One thing that had made me agree to getting married was that through all the difficulties we had so far faced, Jeff had never once mentioned leaving me. Good or bad, he wanted to go through it with me.

Step families are renowned for problems between the new partner and their natural children. Many times the situation doesn't work out, and it is so difficult to overcome the many issues that arise when a stranger comes into the lives of children, and has some of their parents' love. Sometimes I felt Jeff was being unreasonable, sometimes I was thankful that he was there to share things with. Relationships are never perfect, and I don't believe those people who proclaim, "We've never had a cross word." If that were true, they either spend lots of time apart or they are very boring people, in my opinion.

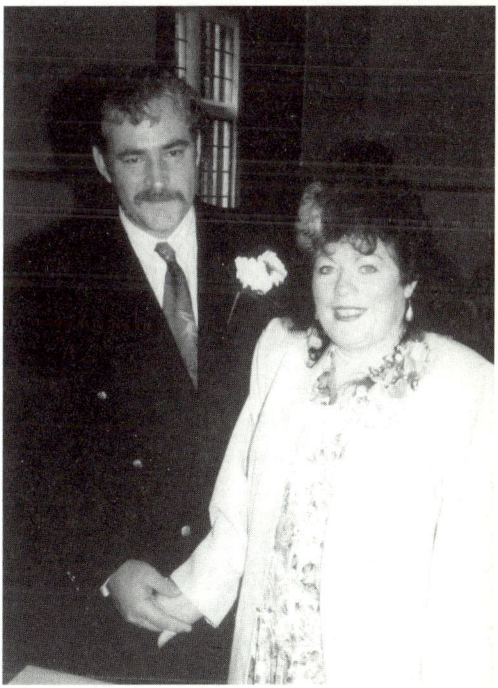

With Jeff on our wedding day, 1994

On our wedding day Emma had obviously called something of a truce. She was lovely and began the day by buying me some flowers. I knew that, despite all the differences between us, she loved me enough to want me to be happy. My family came down to Brighton for the wedding; it was the first time they had seen Emma with her new look. She wore a checked shirt and black trousers and, most importantly to me, she smiled a lot on that day, something she had done so rarely in recent months. Lucy was very happy; she had always got along with Jeff—in fact it is very difficult not to get along with Lucy, she has such a lovely nature. Although she obviously knew that Emma was gay by this time, Lucy didn't really understand what it meant, and consequently she didn't know why it had made such a difference to our family. But she was only eleven years old and had quite enough with all her own problems to contend with.

After the wedding, life carried on much the same. There were good days and bad days between Emma and me. Our disagreements were about the usual things: her staying out late, who she was mixing with, where she was going, and so on. I refused to let her have her girlfriends to stay over, which obviously wouldn't have been the case if she hadn't been gay (in that case, I wouldn't have let her have boyfriends to stay over!).

I suppose some people may think me rather old fashioned in these days when anything goes and is seen as acceptable, but that doesn't worry me, I have values which I believe are right. I can't remember how many times I said to Emma, "While you're living in my house..." to which she would usually walk away. Although she had quite a lot of freedom by this time, Emma was not yet 16, so she was still a child and my responsibility. She loathed it when I reminded her of this, and especially when I ended a telling-off session with the words "my girl"!

In April 1995, a heated argument about Emma not being

allowed to stay over in Brighton with friends ended with me telling her that if she wanted to behave in that way, she would have to leave home. I felt that I couldn't cope any longer with all the worrying and wondering what she was doing; at night when she was out I couldn't sleep until I heard her key in the door and knew she was safely home.

Something had to give, it just couldn't go on. If Emma wanted her freedom, if she wanted to do just what she wanted then she would have to do so away from our home. I had Lucy to consider as well as Emma, and didn't want her life filled with tension and sadness.

I can't tell you, because there are no words, how I felt as Emma slammed the door behind her. It was as though the door had slammed on Emma's childhood, on those days when I had been the centre of her world, when I had fulfilled every need she had. In place of my lovely little girl was this adolescent, arrogant person who was frequently mistaken for a boy, such was her appearance. I could no longer reach her with anything I said because I knew nothing of the way of life she wanted. I knew, though, that she would come up against bigotry and that despite her outer bravado she would suffer.

I had always dreaded the day that my daughters would leave home, but had hoped that it would be when they were old enough, and that they would be leaving in circumstances other than the ones in which Emma left. Emotionally I was not ready to let go of her, and she was not old enough to leave. She had always been headstrong; from when she was very small she would dominate a situation if she could get away with it, and I had always had to be very definite that she should do what she was told, rather than what she wanted. I am in no way condoning her father's lack of patience with her when she was little, but even as young as four or five she would often argue with him until he lost his temper.

It was my fortieth birthday a few days after Emma left, the saddest birthday of my life. I telephoned Sainsbury's to see whether she had turned up for work, and when they said that she had, I knew at least that she was safe.

A few days afterwards, she phoned me and arranged to meet. I was so relieved to hear from her, because I knew she couldn't have much money, and when we met she told me that the other women in the house in which she was living were looking after her. She said that she didn't want to come home, despite my pleas for her to do so. She was of course still considered a minor, not yet being 18, and should things not work out for her living where she was, she could be taken into care by the local authority. It was a truly dreadful time for us all, and I tried to express my feelings in a poem I wrote at the time.

EMMA

I remember the day that you were born
I say to you, as you stifle a yawn
I suffered agony, it's true
They pushed and pulled
Then they handed me you

I remember the day you started school
Me in a state, felt such a fool
Your little chin wobbled
And your tears would start
When you realised we'd be apart

Then on you grew into your teens
Nothing was how it once had been
So unprepared was I for the day
You stood before me
Saying, "Mum, I'm gay"

No words would come and I started to shake
Put my hand to my heart and I felt it break
Then the door slammed closed
And I couldn't have known
How much it would hurt
When my child left home

Now the years have gone by
And you are quite grown
With so much to do and a life of your own
But love knows no boundary
I know this is true
For you are my daughter
And I do so love you

seventeen

HAVING decided not to return home, Emma took a full-time job in Sainsbury's. She didn't stay long in the house in Brighton and was eventually given a room in a hostel for young women in the town. The hostel was run by Social Services, and Emma had a key worker looking after her, which basically meant that she was 'in care'. This really caused me great sadness.

I visited Emma regularly, and she came home every Sunday to have lunch and spend the day. In my wildest dreams I would never have thought that this would happen, but there seemed nothing else that could be done. I knew that Emma was very disappointed in me as her mother because I found it so hard to accept this monumental change in her. But it wasn't just the fact that she was gay—she couldn't help that—I think it was her appearance almost as much as her attitude which was so difficult to accept. Sometimes her hair was almost totally shaved off, and I just couldn't adapt to the masculine dress code she had adopted as quickly as Emma wanted me to. It was as though I was reluctantly having to let go of one Emma and accept this other, very different, Emma.

There was never a week when I didn't phone or visit her, never a day when I didn't wish that she could come home and that things would be well between us all. In real life, however, wishing can be a futile pastime. I told Emma frequently that I loved her so much, and hoped my actions of keeping in close touch with her and visiting her showed her it was true.

The other tenants in the hostel where Emma lived were certainly an eye opener to her: some of them were there because they had been abused, some were there because they were drug addicts, and some were just girls who had been rejected by their families since they were born and consequently had no idea what it meant to be part of a loving family. Although at the time Emma and her family were going through hell, I knew in my heart that the bond we had shared through all the years of her growing up would be strong enough to get us through this awful time. I knew also that Emma's character was very strong and that she would get through this and be stronger for it.

Despite what had happened, it was still my intention to try and get a move to Ashford, as I wanted to be nearer to my family. Emma was adamant that she didn't want to leave Brighton, which was her choice and I couldn't force her. We put an advertisement in a paper, saying that we needed a property which had been adapted for a wheelchair user, and I was most surprised when we had four or five replies. One of these came from a couple who had a house in Swanley, which was some forty minutes away from Ashford; the lady of the house was a multiple sclerosis victim, who was eager to move to the Brighton area. We visited the house, which had three bedrooms and a through-floor lift. I tried the lift, which was situated in the corner of the kitchen and went up into the bedroom. The reason for having a lift such as this rather than a stairlift was to accommodate someone in their wheelchair. Multiple sclerosis is a progressive disease and the council were looking to the future when they installed it, although at the time of our meeting the lady was still able to walk well.

I didn't really like the feeling of claustrophobia I experienced once the lift door had closed, and I felt rather as though I was sitting in a huge microwave oven as I peered through the transparent top half of the door. The roof of the lift was the floor of the bedroom when it was downstairs; as the lift went up into the bedroom, so the floor of the lift became the ceiling of the kitchen.

In practice, these lifts are very ingenious, making it possible for a wheelchair user to live in a house rather than being confined to single storey accommodation. However they do take up a lot of floor space, which is difficult in properties that aren't very large. Although the house was by no means perfect, reality told me that perhaps it was the best option available at the time. I would have liked to have been able to move into a bungalow such as I was leaving in Peacehaven, but bungalows are like gold dust and there aren't too many adapted properties available, so both Jeff and I felt that perhaps we shouldn't pass this chance up.

We moved to Swanley in April 1996, but we only stayed in the house there for nine months or so. We were never happy there, one of the main reasons being that the previous tenants with whom we had swapped had been economical with the truth as regards the neighbours and their two boisterous children, who thought nothing of jumping over the fence into our garden as and when they liked. Lucy wasn't happy at her new school at all, and became very weepy and anxious.

I knew we had made a mistake. Although it took forty minutes to drive to Ashford rather than almost two hours as it had done from Brighton, I didn't see much more of my family. I drove down every Saturday to visit my mother; prior to that time I hadn't had much experience of motorway driving, and unfortunately the infamous M25 was now right on our doorstep and the only way out!

Although I'm not a nervous driver, I must say that initially it put the fear of God into me! There was so much traffic and so many lanes, and if you got into the wrong one on the roundabout before the motorway, you'd had it—you just had to go in that direction. I persevered, however, and became hardened to motorway driving. It was 'every man for himself' on the road and that was how I geared myself up mentally to deal with it.

The one good thing that happened during that time was that I had a voluntary job with a hospice team; I manned the switchboard for the Ellenor Hospice nurses who had an office in Gravesend. Over the few months I was there, I got to know them well. There were about ten nurses, who were based at Gravesend and visited people in the surrounding area who were suffering from cancer. They were helpful to me right from the start, when I went for the interview and found the slope outside the building too steep for me to walk up without anything to lean on. When I told them this they immediately said that they would have a rail put there for me—nothing was too much trouble.

The nurses visited people in their own homes, including babies and young children, and although I was only involved in as much as I was taking messages, it brought home to me what heartache people go through. It had been bad enough losing my father to that dreadful disease, but how I would have coped if one of my babies had cancer I don't know. The Ellenor was not a place in which you could feel sorry for yourself; should you have such a disposition, many of its staff were religious people and I always presumed that it was their faith that gave them the strength it must have taken to do such a job. They had their own chaplain, a young mum also based at the Gravesend office. She became a good friend and I was sorry to leave the Ellenor and all its wonderful staff. I will never forget my time there.

By this time Emma was in a steady relationship. She had met her girlfriend, Landy, while working at Sainsbury's and seemed much happier in herself. She visited us regularly now and I had met Landy a few times. I can't say it was easy, but if she made Emma happy that was all I cared about.

Emma had now left the hostel, and had moved in with Landy's family. I was surprised that Landy's mother was so tolerant of the situation as neither of the girls were 18 yet, but I was thankful to her that Emma was now living somewhere where she was content. Landy was the female side of the relationship and as such, had not cut her hair; to look at her you wouldn't know that she was gay. Although she usually wore jeans she would sometimes wear a skirt, something Emma would rather die than do!

I remember with some humour that when Emma first went to Sainsbury's she was told she would have to wear an overall, black tights and ladies' black shoes. She was horrified at this prospect and had begrudgingly put the overall on, but, ever the rebel, had worn black trousers underneath, as well as her beloved Dr Martens boots and green luminous socks! She looked hilarious and drew far more attention to herself than if she had done as she was told. We laugh about that now, but Emma was so stubborn. Nevertheless, after voicing her objection to skirts, she was allowed to wear trousers.

Although we were not happy in our new home, there was no way the housing association to which it belonged would move us after only living there for a few months. I was determined however, having come this far, that we should move nearer to Ashford and preferably, to a bungalow or single storey accommodation. So I looked into the possibility of private renting, which was really becoming quite a popular and, for the owners, lucrative option now. After telephoning many estate agents in the Ashford area, we finally found a bungalow

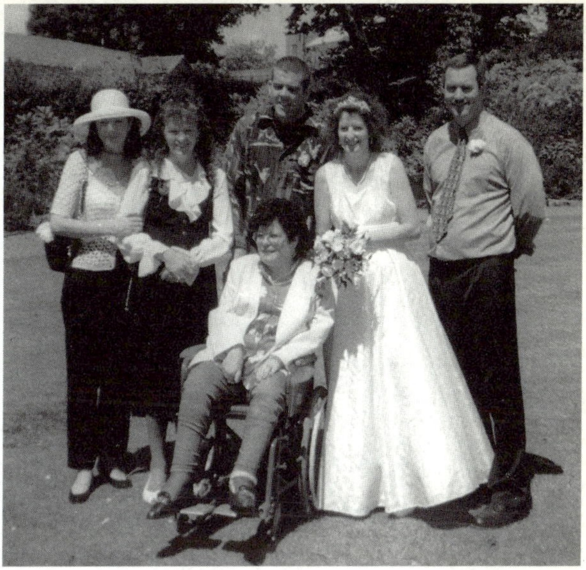

At Anne's wedding, 1998

which was situated quite near to Ashford, just outside Folkestone, and we arranged to go and view it. The rent on the bungalow was £450 per month; because we received income support, part of the rent would be paid for us (though at the time we viewed the property we didn't know how much we would have to pay ourselves).

The bungalow turned out to be set in a beautiful, rural area called 'Walnut Lodge' and had a huge 100 foot long garden surrounded by tall conifers; it was like nothing I had ever lived in before. The landlord was a farmer who lived nearby on his farm, and had bought the bungalow both as an investment and as somewhere he and his wife could live in their retirement. They were a lovely couple in their middle age and we got on very well. It didn't take us long to decide that we would love to live in Walnut Lodge and we could see no reason why we shouldn't live there for many years. Once all the paperwork had been done, it was decided that we would have to pay £100 of the rent per month ourselves and the benefit office would pay the remainder. We did, however, have to put down two months' rent prior to moving in; this came to almost £1000, for which we took out a loan.

Some people may have thought it silly of us to leave a property where we had security and in which we could live rent free, but if you are unhappy in a situation in life and you have the means to get yourself out of that situation, you should do so. Nobody else will do it for you.

We were all happy during our time at Walnut Lodge and never regretted the move. My dog, Squeaker, loved the big garden: it must have felt as though she had a park all to herself! She was ten years old by this time and had developed a cough, which I put down to old age. When Jeff took her to the vet for a routine injection, however, he was told that Squeaker had developed a small heart murmur, but at that stage it wasn't serious.

Lucy settled in to her new school, the Harbour School in nearby Dover. As before, she had a taxi there each day, paid for by the local authority, and from the first time we went to look at the school, I felt it would be more pleasant than the school in Dartford had been. Lucy made friends here and quickly became her happy-go-lucky self.

Once again I looked for some voluntary work and found a job at a hospital in Ashford, working on the outpatients help line. Basically, this was taking calls from people who were not able to attend an appointment, and putting them through to the relevant department to make alternative appointments for them. One of the reasons I had thought about working in a hospital was that obviously the access would be good, and there would be disabled toilets. There are so many things to consider when a disabled person looks for work, and everything has to be just right for their individual requirements, otherwise they can't cope.

I was surprised by the attitude of some of my fellow workers at the hospital. For instance, I needed help to get my chair out of my car. At first it seemed there would be no problem in a porter coming out to the car park and giving me a hand, but in practice it didn't work like that, and when I phoned the porters' lodge there was never anyone available to help me. I was very angry at the attitudes I encountered when asking for help—after all, I was working for nothing but my monthly expenses.

The hospital then purchased an electric wheelchair themselves which I could use and which would be kept at the hospital—so that I would only have to walk in, and the chair would be there. Although the chair itself was fine, they decided that it would have to be kept chained to the stairs, because wheelchairs were always going missing.

Although I agreed in principle with this, it meant that I still had to ask someone to unlock the chain—and I hated asking for help, mainly because of the initial reaction I had encountered. I also felt that certain people had made up their minds as to what I could do rather than ask me. After working on the helpline for a few months, I felt I would like to do something else within the hospital. There was a position going in the switchboard department, so I went down to see the set up. Once it had all been explained to me, I felt that I could manage, making clear that the only problem I could immediately foresee was that I would need my telephone headset put on. I was told that this wasn't a problem and that they would let me know what they decided.

More than six weeks passed and I heard nothing, and when I finally asked the volunteer manager what was happening about the job, he told me that the supervisor of the switchboard department had decided I couldn't manage it. I was so angry, partly because she had not told me what she thought, but also because she had made up her mind what I could do without possibly knowing. Maybe I wouldn't have been able to manage, but I should certainly have been given the chance to find out. Sometimes people are so small-minded that they think if you can't use two hands and do things the way they do them, then it's not possible to do them at all.

That type of person is the kiss of death for disabled people, and I hope the Disabled Discrimination Act, due to come into force in 2005, will do something to stop their damaging attitudes. Because of the general apathy that I felt existed with regard to finding me more challenging work, and because I was not permitted to work with a computer as I wasn't a paid member of staff, I left the hospital after a year or so.

Sadly, we only stayed in Walnut Lodge for just over a year. This was because the landlord's farm was in some financial trouble and he had decided that the only way he could rectify this was to sell the bungalow. We were very sad when this happened and so was he, as his dream of retiring there had been shattered.

We approached the local council in Folkestone, only to be told that we were not eligible for council housing in the area, and that the supply of housing for disabled people was very low. Of course, the fact that we had left secure housing in Swanley of our own volition was also used against us, and all we were offered was a place in a hostel where we could well be indefinitely.

This was a dreadfully worrying time; we only had six weeks or so to vacate Walnut Lodge before it was to be put up for sale, so once again we scoured the local estate agents' advertisements for a suitable bungalow. We had decided that, as we had no other option but to move into privately rented housing again, we might as well look for something in Ashford, which was where we had set out to move originally.

We had spent a few fruitless weeks searching when my mother phoned me, saying that she had seen a bungalow advertised which was situated near Ashford town centre. I immediately made arrangements with the estate agent to view the bungalow, but was initially told that the landlord wasn't keen on having tenants who received income support. I suspected this was because, unfortunately, people often tar everyone with the same brush, thinking that if you receive income support it is because you are too lazy to go to work.

I put this view over to the estate agent, who duly explained our circumstances to the landlord. Ironically enough, he turned out to be disabled himself and was quite happy to have us as tenants. On the way to the viewing, the estate agent mentioned almost in passing that the bungalow had 'a couple of steps' down to it. I was horrified at this news, knowing that it would make all the difference as to whether or not we could live there. The 'couple' of steps turned out to be three huge steps, which I would never be able to manage, and I could see that it would also be difficult to ramp them because they were quite steep.

However, there was a grass bank down one side of the steps which I used to gain access on our initial visit into the bungalow; and apart from the fact that it was rather small for a wheelchair user, the bungalow was suitable for our needs. It had two bedrooms, a huge lounge and very small kitchen and bathroom. Whilst the social services were happy to discuss putting a ramp down for me, they wouldn't visit until we had moved in; that was their policy, and however much I pointed out that we couldn't move in without a ramp being in place, it made no difference.

Although I had managed to get my wheelchair down the grass bank, it was only because the grass was dry at the time, and there was no way I could do that in the winter months. After exploring every avenue for help it became clear that if we wanted to live in the bungalow, we would have to supply the ramp ourselves. After discussing the options available as to what materials would be best to use for the ramp, we eventually decided that concrete would be safest. We didn't know how long we might live in this bungalow. That's the thing with renting someone else's property—you never know when you'll have to vacate it.

However, whether we lived there for three months or three years I still needed the ramp, which cost us £700, paid for weekly over 18 months with a Social Security loan. By now I had an electric hoist fitted into the back of my Metro, which lifted my electric wheelchair into the car. This gave me far greater freedom, and enabled Lucy and me to go out on our own. The hoist had been fitted by David Hodge, the grandson of my original engineer, who had retired some years before. My wheelchair has to be partially taken apart in order for it to fit into the back of my car, which means that I can't do it independently. This is something I find very frustrating, and I look forward to the time when I have a larger car, when I will be able to do this unaided and have total freedom to come and go as I please.

It was during the time we were living in the bungalow in Ashford that our beloved dog Squeaker became very ill. Her heart murmur, which had been diagnosed over two years previously, had steadily become worse. She started to cough as her lungs took in fluid, because her heart had become enlarged and was not working properly. By the time she died she was taking more than 6 tablets a day, and it was so difficult to get them into her. We tried putting them in her food, but she was very crafty and after a while she would leave them in her bowl. We tried giving them to her between slices of chicken roll, ham, chocolate, cake, biscuits—you name it, we tried it! Of course, when she had been on her medication for a year or so, its effectiveness lessened and she was coughing despite it.

Eventually she began to leave wet patches where she sat, which she found distressing as she was a very clean dog. It was so difficult to come to terms with the fact that Squeaker's life had to come to an end, and more difficult to be the one who had to make the decision that it was time she should be put to sleep. We had had her in the family for almost thirteen years and, needless to say, we adored her.

Emma and Lucy had grown up with Squeaker; and for me, during some very lonely difficult periods of my life, she had always been there, sitting beside me and giving me such comfort. If I was ever upset, she would look up at me and, putting her head on my lap, push my arm out of the way with her nose, because she knew I couldn't move my arm myself. Losing her was too difficult to contemplate, but she had given me such love and been so loyal throughout her precious life that I owed it to her not to let her suffer or to lose her dignity.

The vet came to our home by request. It was a truly dreadful day, the day of the eclipse, and seemed surreal; even though it was morning it seemed more like dusk, and everywhere was strangely quiet. I thought it a fitting atmosphere for such a sad day. Lucy and I said goodbye to Squeaker in our garden before Jeff took her indoors and was with her at the end. As much as I wanted to be there, I could not bear to witness it. Jeff was so strong for us all that day.

We had Squeaker cremated, and we keep her ashes on the mantelpiece in a little box inscribed 'Our Sunshine Girl', because she loved the sun and basking in the warm shadows it made on the carpet. Some people may not understand such strength of feeling for an animal, but anyone who has ever loved a dog certainly will.

eighteen

AFTER living in the bungalow for just over a year, we were finally offered a house by Ashford Council. We were so relieved that at last we would have some security in our home, and not have to wonder how long we could stay there.

The house had previously been lived in by a wheelchair user and so was already adapted, with level access and a through-floor lift. I'm not keen on the lift, but I hope that in time my preference for a stair lift might be acted upon by the Council.

The bath had a seat that lifts up and down enabling me to have a bath independently, which is so important. The kitchen is very spacious, with low level cupboards and room to turn a wheelchair round without bumping into things, which I find so frustrating! Knowing at first hand how expensive these modifications are, we didn't look the gift horse in the mouth, and accepted the offer immediately.

The house had been empty for some six months because other prospective tenants were not keen on having the lift. But everything comes down to money and Ashford Council were adamant that they would not remove it in favour of a stairlift while it was still in working order.

I know that if you turn down a suitable property without good reason you are likely to be put to the back of the queue, and unfortunately adapted properties are few and far between in most local authorities. Ideally I would always prefer to live in a bungalow rather than a house, as it gives me a feeling of security that I don't have when living in a place with an upstairs, but like most things in life, after a time I get used to it.

The lift was a bit of a worry for me in the first few months that I lived in the house as it had been standing idle for a long time and was rather temperamental! It would either stop halfway between floors or, when it had arrived at its destination, the doors wouldn't open. Because I suffer from claustrophobia, I found using the lift very worrying initially, but as there was no other way for me to get upstairs I had no choice but to get on with it.

We have lived here for over two years, and now also have a stairlift. We are very happy in our home, and feel we have finally achieved our goal; it has cost us a great deal of money with renting privately, but there was no other way to do it. I see my family regularly now and it is good to be here where I was born 45 years ago. So much has happened to me in those years: I have known great sadness, especially as a child; but I have also known times of great triumph, such as when I had my children and proved, most importantly to myself, that I could care for them; and when I first drove a car.

I have watched my dear Lucy grow from that tiny scrap of humanity into the lovely young woman she is today, she has just celebrated her 19th birthday and is now working at Woolworth's, where she is given the support she needs. I am truly proud of Lucy. I know that sometimes she finds things very difficult to understand and remember, but she is a fighter and is determined to overcome her problems. I never forget how much worse things could so easily have been for Lucy, given how premature she was. She is a star.

Emma is now 23 years old. She is a compassionate woman who, not surprisingly, feels very confident among disabled

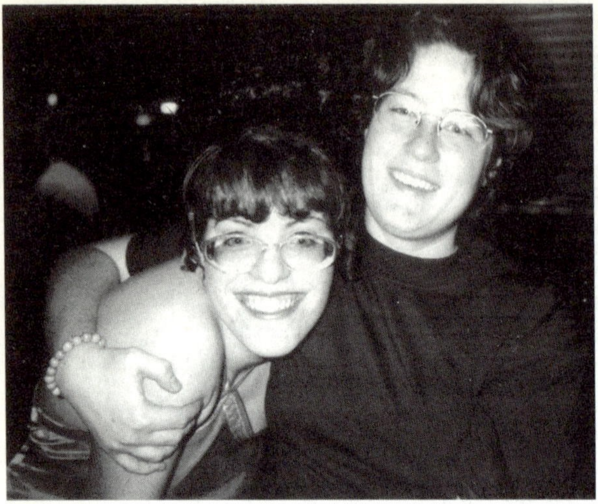

Lucy & Emma, Lucy's 18th birthday

people, and she has a great deal of personal experience with which to help them. Her first relationship lasted for four years, and although she was devastated when it ended, she has great inner strength which helped her through her pain.

Two years ago, Emma became interested in the Buddhist faith and, after learning something of their ways, she decided to become ordained. Since her ordination, she is now known by everyone as Gawa, which means 'one of great joy'. However, in spite of my acceptance of her wishes, I cannot call her by anything other than the name I gave her, and she is quite understanding of that. Emma now lives in a Buddhist commune near Brighton. She has become very devout and her beliefs are everything to her. She wears robes and her head is completely shaved, as is the custom of Buddhist nuns. She still works as a carer and finds great contentment in her life.

When she told me what she wanted to do with her life, I gave her my blessing, as I really want my children to find happiness wherever they can. I confess that, if it were my choice, I would not wish Emma to go down the path she has chosen, as despite my attempts otherwise, I cannot help but feel that I have somehow lost her. Selfishly, I would far rather she lived nearby and was a mum with whom I could share children and all the other things that mums and grownup daughters share. But it is not our place as parents to dictate what lives our precious children live; rather it is our task is to bring them up as well as we can, and set them on the road to life with as good a preparation as we know how to give. I am loved very much by Emma, and that is certainly more important to me than anything else.

Emma visits us often and I am confident that the closeness which bonded us in her childhood years will be there always. Both my children are the greatest joy of my life; I consider it a privilege to be their mother.

Although as a family we agree that Squeaker was irreplaceable, we now have another dog. Ruby is also a Staffordshire bull terrier, but unlike Squeaker has not known love and kindness throughout her life; she is a rescue dog some six years old. Her character is more outgoing than Squeaker's, and she is more nervous and easily startled by noises, which causes her to bark like mad and go round in circles until one of us can calm her down! We have had Ruby for almost two years now. In the first few months I wasn't sure that we had done the right thing in getting her, but she has settled down now and it gives me a good feeling to know that as a family we have given a home to an animal whose life had not been happy. I take her out every day and she walks very well beside my wheelchair, on to which I tie her lead.

Something that I have developed a keen interest in over the last few years is gardening. I have always grown plants in containers and tended them in the parts of the garden I have had access to in my wheelchair, but I had never before had a garden that was completely suited to my needs. I was really delighted, therefore, when I came across an organisation called Gardening For The Disabled Trust. What they do, after a preliminary visit and confirmation of the person's disability by doctor's letter, is to give a grant of £600 so that the disabled person can have their garden made more suitable for their particular need. In my case, I had all grass removed and replaced by a paved area, so that I can get into the garden even after it has been raining and not have to worry about muddy wheels.

I find it really rewarding to see the garden looking bright and colourful, knowing that I have been able to plant it myself. I am able to water the garden independently by using a hose that is stored on a reel. When I want to use it, I place the head of the hose between my knees and as I move my wheelchair around the garden, so the hose unwinds—simple really! I think it is so important to have interests in life, and it can be very fulfilling.

I have been working at the Wheelchair Users Group for the past two years. This is a charity based in Folkestone which provides disabled people and their carers with information on a wide range of subjects, including where and how to find the best wheelchair for a person's individual needs, holidays, work, benefits and housing, from information we have on our database. We also operate schemes in which we loan people wheelchairs and powered scooters on a long term basis, as well as helping people who need wheelchairs for short periods of time—if they have broken their leg, for instance. We have a membership of some thousand people in the south east Kent area who all receive our quarterly magazine *Wheel Power*, which contains information and articles, some of which are written by our members.

I am the membership secretary and work with the Chairman, Allen Jones, who is a wheelchair user, disabled by muscular dystrophy. Allen founded the Group in 1993 and works very hard to help disabled people. He has great understanding of their needs and cares about what happens to them, always ensuring that he provides them with the right equipment.

Over the years he has come to be greatly respected by many people and agencies with whom his work brings him into contact, such as Social Services and local authority groups. We work very well together and enjoy a good sense of humour, which is essential in the work we do. The Wheelchair Users Group also has a support helpline, from which people can get both practical and emotional support.

For my part I am glad to have something in my life which gives me the opportunity to help other people, some of whom are newly disabled, either because they are elderly or because they may have been involved in some kind of accident. Whatever the cause, people often think it is the end of the world because they cannot function in the way they used to. Many of them have no idea what help they can get, financial or practical, and I find it very satisfying to inform them about things which I know will make their lives easier.

Although Allen and I run the Wheelchair Users Group together, we work very closely with disability information services, whose office is next door to ours, often passing clients over to one another depending on what help they need. When people come into the office and see that the people who run it are themselves wheelchair users, it gives them the comfort of knowing that we understand their problems, because we've probably come across them ourselves. Thus we never hear the phrase "You don't understand"! It also seems to give some purpose to our disabilities, that we have overcome so much for a reason. Knowledge is power, and it is a good thing to be able to pass it on to others. It is said that adversity introduces us to ourselves; I think these words are absolutely true.

I wanted to write this book for many reasons. To document how I managed to deal with many practical problems was important to me, because if I only help one person with theirs, it will have been worth writing it. But I'd like to think that my experiences may help many people; that when they have read my story they may be encouraged to be strong and strive for what they want to achieve, no matter how impossible it seems or what other people say, whether doubting their capabilities or killing them with kindness.

It seems to me that the key to achievement and independence is within us and we ourselves have to believe that we can attain it. I hope it will help disabled people feel that, just because their bodies don't work in the same way that 'normal' people's bodies do, it doesn't make them any less worthy as people, and they mustn't ever let anyone make them feel that way.

I am sure that, as has happened in the last twenty years or so (before which time a disabled toilet was virtually unheard of), society will continue to become more and more accepting of disabled people. I notice such a difference now in the way I am treated by people than I was twenty-five years ago: for instance, when I'm out in the park with my dog, children look at my face and often say "hello" rather than just staring at my wheelchair as they would have done years ago. There doesn't seem to be the same stigma attached to a disabled person, and terms such as 'spastic' don't seem to be bandied about as an insult in the way that they used to be.

Public places such as pubs, cinemas, restaurants and libraries have far better access for wheelchair users, so that when we go out we don't have to make special arrangements. Having to do this, in itself, always makes you feel different from other people.

Of course, there is always room for improvement and there is a lot more to be done, but because schools like Chailey Heritage, where disabled children were put all together out in a very rural setting, have now generally gone and been replaced by establishments where integration and day boarding are the norm, children don't experience the same feelings of isolation that I did. It's also far more usual now for disabled children to be integrated into mainstream schools which adapt their premises for wheelchair users when possible, so that both the disabled child and the able-bodied children can accept one another from an early age, and by the time they reach adolescence, disability is part and parcel of their lives.

I think it is very important for disabled people to be portrayed in more positive ways, especially by the media. For example, if disabled people were more commonplace in soap operas, and their day-to-day struggles were discussed in everyday situations, it would help people to understand that disabled people are just, as I have said before, people with disabilities. It may also help to eliminate some of the fear and embarrassment that some able-bodied people feel when they come across a disabled person.

There will always be those members of society who shun disabled people; always a few who think that because you have a physical disability you must be feeble-minded as well. But it is they who are feeble-minded, with their unenlightened view that because someone is using a wheelchair, or not able to hear or speak in the 'normal' way, they can't be accepted by society and treated as worthy human beings. My hope is that these people are few and far between, and become more so; and that disabled people will continue to be integrated more and more in society, as the architectural barriers come down and we can access anywhere we choose.

We may have a long way to go, and the journey may at times seem never ending, but it's sometimes worth looking over our shoulder and seeing just how far we've come.

With the girls... (sisters Anne, Catherine and Lynne)

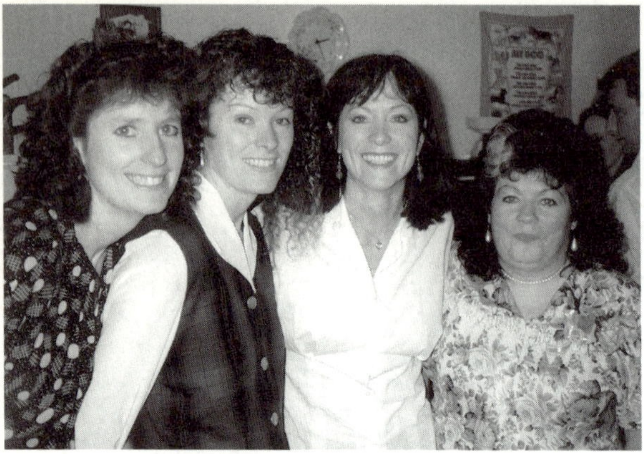

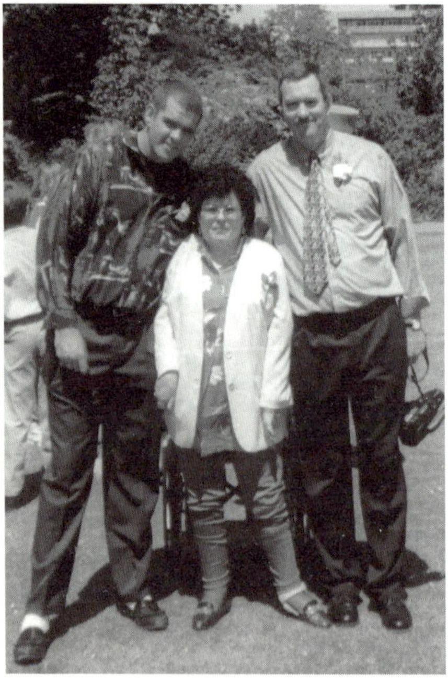

...and the boys! (brothers Davy Joe and Willie James)

About the author

Maureen Fenner was born in 1955 in Ashford in south-east Kent. She contracted polio at the age of three months and as a result both of her arms and her left hand were paralysed. She also lost most of the use of her right hand and her legs were severely weakened by the virus.

From the age of three to sixteen years she was educated and cared for at Chailey Heritage, a specialised school in East Sussex which also provided clinical and medical care.

Maureen learned to type with the use of an adapted typewriter and secured secretarial work both in her home town of Ashford and then in Brighton on the south coast. She married and had two children: Emma, born in 1978, and Lucy, born prematurely in 1982 weighing only 1lb 13ozs.

Maureen currently lives in Ashford with her husband Jeff, her daughter Lucy, and Ruby, her Staffordshire bull terrier. She is a member of the British Polio Fellowship and works part-time for the Wheelchair Users Group in Folkestone.

For more information about our
publications, please write to:

Heartland Publishing Limited
P.O.Box 902, Sutton Valence
Maidstone, Kent ME17 3HY

or email: publish@heartland.co.uk